The Rules of Radiology

Paul McCoubrie

The Rules of Radiology

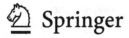 Springer

Paul McCoubrie
North Bristol NHS Trust
Bristol, UK

ISBN 978-3-030-65231-9   ISBN 978-3-030-65229-6   (eBook)
https://doi.org/10.1007/978-3-030-65229-6

This Springer imprint is published by the registered company Springer Nature Switzerland AG
The registered company address is: Gewerbestrasse 11, 6330 Cham, Switzerland

To my lovely prize-winning author wife, Rachel, for her support, tolerance, and damn fine editing skills. This book wouldn't be in your hands without her.

Preface

Hello and welcome to this book.

If you have bought this book then you are either a radiologist or someone who is interested in radiology. Or possibly my mother (Hi Mum!). Irrespective of who you are, hopefully you'll find much in the following pages that will be directly relevant to your personal and professional life. It may even raise a dry smile: Lord knows that those have been in short supply recently.

This book addresses what I see as the most important issues in radiology. To be specific, it takes a critical look at the day-to-day practice of radiology and teases out the important bits. Not always the popular or topical bits, but the nitty-gritty of what radiology is actually all about. These are the topics that radiologists know intuitively but actually rarely discuss. I explain why these topics are so important and should be discussed.

It isn't a textbook by any stretch of the imagination; there are plenty of those already. Nor is it a manifesto; I'm no politician. It isn't just a critical look at the world of radiology but it gives considered guidance about how radiologists and others can not only survive but also thrive amidst the tricky modern medical world.

In that respect, it is a letter to my younger self. Apart from saying, "sit down, shut up and get a haircut", this overlong letter contains all of the scraps of wisdom I've gathered thus far in my time on this planet. By presenting these as Rules to be obeyed, it makes up an unofficial curriculum for young radiologists starting out into the world. For others it provides a reality check; a mirror to hold themselves up against. It is an extensive critique of modern radiology but it also conveys a valuable message of hope in these turbulent times.

You will note that this book deals with Rules of Radiology #1-50 but there are multiple references to Rules #51-100. These are listed in Appendix 1. My intention is write a second volume to cover Rules #51-100. However, I am contractually obliged to not do so for a year from the publication date of this book otherwise my wife says she will probably leave me. Given that I'm rather fond of her, you will have to wait for the second volume, I am afraid. But hopefully it will be worth the wait.

Bristol, UK   Paul McCoubrie

Acknowledgements All the artwork are original pieces by John Charlesworth, my immensely talented Uncle. Many thanks to him.

Several individuals have offered support and constructive comments. I'd particularly like to thank Barry Kelly but also Adrian Brady, Giles Maskell, Philip Ward, Guy Burkill, and last but not least, my father, Malcolm McCoubrie.

Contents

Chapter 1
Rule #1 / / Obey The Rules

Your reason is to knowingly breach The Rules isn't good enough. It never will be. It is also forbidden for someone familiar with The Rules to knowingly assist another person to breach them.

—

The average reader will look at the introductory paragraph and be slightly baffled. Of all the medical specialities, why does radiology need Rules? And why do radiologists have to obey them? Furthermore, why do radiologists have to insist that others obey the Rules in a similarly rigid fashion? And more to the point, who is this McCoubrie chap and why the hell does he think he can tell others what to do? So many questions, such anger, such perplexity.

Before anything else, I should point out The Rules are my opinions. They aren't a legal document. I'm not going to instruct counsel to prosecute you in the event of a transgression. But if you don't obey The Rules then I will do what all right-thinking Britons do when severely provoked. I will fix you with a hard stare and tut quietly.

The other thing is The Rules is predominantly a work of satire. You may quote them freely but they aren't evidence-based or in any way binding. So, for God's sake, don't quote me in anything serious. I'm not appearing as an Expert Witness on the back of one of my assertions. But I am being perfectly serious in my satirical aims. My goal is to first make you laugh then make you think. As George Bernard Shaw once wrote, 'My method is to take the utmost trouble to find the right thing to say, and then to say it with the utmost levity'.

By way of introduction, I'm a middle-aged male white British radiologist (Fig. 1.1). I've specifically tried to avoid any cultural bias but if some unconscious bias has crept in, I apologise. This said, The Rules apply to all radiologists irrespective of age, gender, cultural heritage or country of residence.

The book is about radiology. Not radiotherapy or anything to do with radios. If you aren't medical, radiology is sometimes known as the 'X-ray department',

© The Author(s), under exclusive license to Springer Nature Switzerland AG 2021
P. McCoubrie, *The Rules of Radiology*, https://doi.org/10.1007/978-3-030-65229-6_1

Fig. 1.1 "By way of
introduction, I'm a middle-
aged male white radiologist"

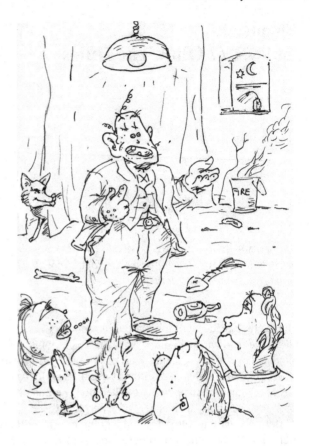

'roentgenography' (only in the US) or the loathsome 'medical imaging'.
Radiology is a post-graduate medical speciality. Like Anaesthetists, patients are
often surprised that we are doctors and not some technically-trained Surgeon's
handmaiden.

Admittedly I am writing about it from a medical perspective but The Rules
equally apply to those involved in working closely with radiologists. There are
many members of the radiology team. The most numerous of which are radiographers (in the UK) but elsewhere they are 'radiology technicians' or similar.
Radiologists work very closely with radiographers. The two trades are interde-
pendent. Radiographers explicitly have to obey The Rules too.

I can reassure you that The Rules have been thoroughly thought through. They
are formed from over twenty years as a radiologist and considerable introspection.
They are also formed from listening to people a lot more intelligent than me and
then stealing their ideas.

Like *La Gaza Lardra* (The Thieving Magpie), I have rapaciously collected the
sparkling wit and collective wisdom of the Great and Good of Radiology. I've

taken old radiological maxims, heuristics, and aphorisms then buffed them up, ready for general viewing. I even wrote quite a few myself.

This isn't a radiology textbook, you will be reassured to hear. There is very little in here about the day-to-day interpretational aspect of the job. I'm not here to spout about how to read X-rays or CT scans. Plenty of people have done this already. This is about the other 50%. The bits of a radiologist's job that isn't look-ing at black and white pictures. Like talking to other doctors. And occasionally patients too.

Okay, I hear you say. It is a book of radiology axioms. With clever-clever words to explain them. But why present them as Rules that must be obeyed? That is a more complex question that will take a little explanation.

Firstly, radiology is different to most forms of medical practice. All the old adages don't translate to our way of working. This is largely because we have his-torically been 'back room' doctors. Radiologists, like pathologists, are largely the 'doctor's doctor'. Our primary goal is to help the patient by helping their doctor. But unlike pathologists and other back-of-house staff, radiology is increasingly front-line and patient-facing. We still help the patient's doctor but we have a public face too.

Secondly, radiology is increasingly homogenous. Rather being cultural-ly-driven, radiology is technically-driven. And in the modern global economy, the technology is the same the world over. Naturally the health systems in each coun-try vary hugely. In some countries there are several different health systems. The number of scanners and access to them varies widely. And the precise numbers of staff, training of the staff, the background of the staff, the style of employment of the staff varies hugely. But a scanner is a scanner. The machines are the same whether they be in Tipperary or Timbuktu.

It is this common technology that binds the global radiology community together like glue. We speak a global radiological language. Day-to-day radiologi-cal practice is remarkably similar the world over. A fully trained radiologist from, say, Manchester would find themselves eminently employable in Moscow and Manila alike.

Thirdly, radiology is in a state of flux and needs direction. It is a massively changing speciality, almost unrecognisable from the speciality I entered over twenty years ago. I don't think any other speciality has seen either such fundamen-tal changes in its practice or such huge growth. And it doesn't show any signs of slowing. I suspect radiology in 2040 will be quite, quite different again.

Half of the procedures that I did as a new consultant radiologist no longer exist. I admit that I miss some of these very dearly. The beautiful simplicity of an intra-venous urogram, done properly, is a thing of singular beauty. If Shakespeare had lived in modern times I am sure he would have written sonnets about the graceful curves of the calyceal system.

Some of these procedures, I must admit that I don't miss at all. And if you asked them, neither would the patients that had to endure them. Lower limb veno-grams and barium enemas were not far off being instruments of medieval torture.

They firmly belong upon the dungheap of medical history. The only thing worth writing about them is laws to ban them ever coming back.

But perhaps the biggest change is massive expansion of cross-sectional imaging. I remember the scanner appeals of the 1980s, where each hospital faced the uphill battle of funding their first CT scanner. Only twenty years ago, MRI scanners were rare beasts; space-age tech that us mere mortals rarely got to see close up. As a very young radiologist, I might have drooled once or twice, such was my slack jawed wonder.

These days each hospital has several of each type of scanner. And they are much, much faster. It takes longer for the patient to clamber into the saddle of the scanner than the ride itself. Twenty years ago it was very very different. On a good day we would scan fifteen patients in CT and be working flat out; now it is more like four to five times that. Back then CT scanners were slower than MRI is now. MRI was glacially slow and the images were murky smears, more like an abstract painting than a depiction of human anatomy.

Lastly, and perhaps most importantly, most mainstream radiology practice makes sense to the casual observer. But when such practice is critically examined, it is often found on to be based on rather shaky logic. Just occasionally current practice makes no sense and is actually counter-productive. For example, many hospitals are now waking up to the fact that the radiologist looking at the most complex scans on the sickest patients needs quiet uninterrupted thinking time. Whereas this couldn't be further from what actually happens.

So. We have established several facts. Radiology needs Rules as it is doesn't already have them; it is different from mainstream medical practice; it is a increasingly homogeneous on a global scale; it is changing so rapidly and much of our practice doesn't bear close inspection.

But you might still be asking about such strict adherence to arbitrary Rules. I don't blame you. Most folk don't like being told what to do. And doctors are particularly fond of their clinical autonomy. The classic notion of persuading a group of doctors to behave uniformly is like trying to herd cats.

So, why should you obey The Rules. It isn't a case of 'I know best, listen to me'. That isn't my style at all. The reason is fairly simple. Read them. Read them all. Then, after due consideration, decide if you agree. And if you do agree, you must obey Rule #1.

Chapter 2
Rule #2 / / Smile

Those who complain the most, accomplish the least. And remember, nobody likes a whinger.

—

There is an saying that it takes forty-three muscles to frown but only seventeen to smile. There is a lesser-known misanthropic addition which points out that it takes just four muscles to slap the smart-arse who comes up with annoying sayings.

The point is that smiling is supposed to be simpler than frowning. Except this isn't necessarily true. When the whole face animates with a full beaming and radiant smile, it often involves all forty-three facial muscles. Yet only six muscles are needed for quite respectable frown. To make matters more complex, you need just four muscles for a rictus grin (left and right *risorius* and *zygomaticus*). And if we are to follow the argument through to the end, a proper slap actually involves around fifty six muscles.

You might think I am missing the point through anatomical pedantry. But radiologists tend to be pedantic. I'm not apologising for this; pedants don't apologise. They just pity the less pedantic individual. They know the warm glow of superiority and truly wish others could have it too, if only they would apply themselves a little more. Plus, if I know my target audience, they'll welcome a brief discussion on the complexity of physical exertion in differing forms of non-verbal communication.

Anyway, this Rule is to encourage cheerfulness *en generale* and discourage moaning. At this point, several questions might arise in your mind. Most pertinent is why should radiologists be cheerful? They aren't paid to be happy. They are here to get on with reporting scans and so forth. You may agree that cheerfulness is a Good Thing. But you may argue that, given the pressures most radiologists are under, being cheerful is distinctly difficult. You might also point out that some individuals are by their very nature dour and that persuading them to be cheerful is a forlorn exercise. And lastly, you might argue that blowing off a bit of steam and having a moan to a colleague is highly therapeutic.

© The Author(s), under exclusive license to Springer Nature Switzerland AG 2021
P. McCoubrie, *The Rules of Radiology*, https://doi.org/10.1007/978-3-030-65229-6_2

I will hopefully persuade you that these questions have answers. Yes, radiologists should be cheerful and that there are many very good reasons for this. Not only that but anyone can do it, even the most miserable sod. And also that having a proper moan is probably the worst thing you can do. Let me explain by painting you a few verbal pictures of grumpy personality types that can be found in radiology departments.

The first is the 'Marvin'. Marvin was a robot with 'a brain the size of a planet', from the *Hitchhiker's Guide to the Galaxy* series. Marvin was labelled a 'paranoid android' but wasn't actually paranoid. He was, however, the personification of pessimism. Marvins are useless colleagues—their negativity stops any activity dead in its tracks. They are emotional black holes that drain all the fun, all the humour, all the life out of anyone or any situation. Their constant moaning and grumbling is grinding. They are very difficult colleagues to be around.

On the other end of the spectrum of sullenness, I introduce my second character, the 'House'. Named after the fictional character 'Dr. Gregory House' in the eponymous series, these individuals are curmudgeonly arses. The fictional Dr. House was a flawed genius, a nonconformist who spoke the truth and didn't care what people thought. I should point out that fictional characters are quite different to real-life colleagues. Lovable and endearing grumpiness is far more attractive on screen than in reality. The day-to-day lack of social graces and endless biting sarcasm grates on the nerves, completely outweighing any occasional stroke of genius.

The last character in this gloomy pantheon is the 'Psychopath'. These radiologists give our sainted profession a bad name as they are the bane of a junior doctor's life. I'll give an example. When I was a young doctor, my boss always wanted his scans performed by a particular radiologist. It was my job to get the scans organised. This involved regular trips to the radiology department to find this particular volatile radiologist. I never knew what mood he would be in. Sometimes, I knocked on his door and he would effusively call, "Ah, come in my dear boy, how can I help". Sometimes, I knocked and before I could utter a word, he screamed "Get out! Get out! Out! Out!".

These unpredictable characters are usually unrepentant about anger-management issues. Even when challenged about their unacceptable behaviour, they blame others. The alarming thing is that such behaviour is tolerated. It is tolerated as these attacks of social incontinence aren't witnessed by the appropriate people. These characters are often sweetness and light to their senior colleagues. They reserve their episodic sociopathic behaviour for those lower down the medical hierarchy.

Having summarised this grouchy group of characters, I hope you don't recognise too many of these characteristics in yourself. And if you do, I hope you are admonished. They aren't flattering. I suspect that you'll recognise traits amongst your current or former colleagues.

It is very important that you don't tackle their behaviour head on. This leads to a World of Pain. Part of being socially incompetent is that you fail to recognise the problem, overestimate your own abilities and don't recognise those same skills in others. It is called the Kruger-Dunning effect. Tackling them doesn't work; they deny the problem and often fight back. Save your energy.

I would advise treating these individuals as 'Time Thieves'. I've found it a very useful way of protecting myself from the antisocial antics of particularly toxic individuals. You will be all too aware that you only have so many hours, minutes and seconds on this planet. You will be all too aware of wanting not to waste this time. You will, in fact, be specifically keen on spending time doing life-affirming and joyous things. A Time Thief steals your time and gives nothing back. Every precious second in their company is one you cannot get back.

Thus you should insulate yourself from these people. Spend the absolute minimum of time in their company. And don't give them a second thought. Cut off any emotion, thoughts, or worries. By doing this, you don't waste time thinking about them either. Try it; you'll thank me afterwards.

But let us focus on the positive message of this Rule. Let's look at the benefits of smiling and acting cheerful.

First off, cheerfulness benefits you as an individual. Any therapist will tell you that if you behave in a cheerful fashion, you feel more cheerful still. That is, pretending to be cheerful actually works. If you deliberately employ cheery words, deeds and actions then you feel happier. The reverse is true. Giving voice to a tirade of negativity actually makes you feel worse. Negative body posture and facial expressions reinforce the misery. Thus moaning and whingeing is something to be avoided at all costs. If you find yourself starting, just stop. Sit up straight, put your shoulders back and force a smile. It is curiously effective.

Before long, you'll find yourself happier. This is a goal in itself. We know that happiness in a radiologist is associated with several positive outcomes. Happy radiologists are productive radiologists. Happy radiologists are healthier. Happy radiologists are less likely to burnout or retire early. No one knows if happier radiologists make fewer mistakes but I'd wager that is true too.

Cheerfulness also benefits those around you. For a radiologist, this is most often your colleagues and other members of the radiology department. And patients like a smiling doctor too. Happy patients and happy staff are the markers of a well-functioning department. A well-functioning department is a good place to work; it can recruit and retain staff, it is popular with clinical colleagues and standards are generally high.

But being cheerful isn't always easy and sometimes you have to pretend. You might want to take the request card being proffered by an interloping clinician and insert it forcibly up their least favourite orifice. But instead, you should force a smile and say, "Sure, no problem. Leave it with me".

This ability to remain cheerful in the face of adversity is not something that comes naturally. Well, there are some folk that are curiously pathologically happy. I suspect them of having being dropped on their head as a child. The rest of us normal mortals have to learn it as a skill. And it all starts with a smile. Practice smiling when you least feel like it and, before you know it, your life and that of those around you will have improved immeasurably.

Chapter 3
Rule #3 / / Keep Your Cool

Losing your temper always makes things worse. Anger reveals weakness of character. Equanimity is hard but worth it.

——

This Rule is the corollary of Rule #2. This Rule additionally demands that a radiologist should not lose their rag: they should be phlegmatic not choleric.

You may well laugh and think that I am just posturing. Maybe I am a little but I rarely lose my temper in the workplace. Like many, I've been sorely tested and failed to hide my irritation. I've been irked by thoughtlessness and failed to conceal my exasperation. But I've never descended to a bestial level; I've never shouted, I've never lost control at work.

This is quite deliberate, quite intentional. As my family will tell you, I'm not naturally imbued with calmness. I suspect that one's spouse and offspring are quite different to work colleagues. They know exactly which buttons to press and which raw nerves to tweak. And like a Skinnerian rat pressing a button for a pellet of food, they cannot help themselves, impulsively poking until their spouse/parent explodes.

I strive for calmness in the workplace and advocate the same for very simple reasons. Firstly, like most unspoken goals in life, I've been influenced by both negative and positive role models. I've encountered some needlessly aggressive senior doctors: I swore would be nothing like them. I also encountered some particularly calm and stoical senior doctors: I swore I would strive to be more like them.

I advocate this as I realised that not everyone shared my passion. Indeed, I've encountered modern-day radiologists who had no filter, no check to their words or emotions. They feel it completely acceptable to flip mid sentence from an austere Abraham Lincoln to a raging Genghis Khan. Sometimes the slight was real, sometimes perceived. Nevertheless, they'd be off. All toys out of the cot and the dummy spat. A gratuitous overreaction.

© The Author(s), under exclusive license to Springer Nature Switzerland AG 2021
P. McCoubrie, *The Rules of Radiology*, https://doi.org/10.1007/978-3-030-65229-6_3

The raging radiologist is totally blind. They completely fail to appreciate the destructive effect on other people and their feelings. They completely fail to appreciate that everyone thinks they are a complete and utter prat.

I've met many radiologists who have clear gambits to avoid such spiralling rage. Some recognise the surge of adrenaline but physically divert themselves into a displacement behaviour. Some feel the pupils and nostrils dilate but mentally pull themselves up short, pause to mentally rearrange themselves, and continue calmly. Some turn their emotional excitement into humour.

Now turning potential anger into humour can work but is a risky strategy. The best strategy I've seen uses the heightened state to channel a particular self-effacing humour. This gambit is successful as the focus of the joke is moved onto the radiologist. It is non-threatening; a serious point can be made humorously and no one gets upset.

Another strategy that can occasionally work is the comedic rant at a third party not present in the room. This third party can be a single person, a group or even a concept. The only way this works is to point out something wrong: an injustice, something ludicrous or an amusing paradox. Berating something or someone that is innocent makes you look bitter and jealous. When fluent and lucid this technique can be funny and constructive. But it is very risky. It is a fine line between an sparklingly fluent critique and a fulminant spitting tirade.

The worst strategy I've seen turns the focus of the humour onto a specific individual that is present. This doesn't work. It always belittles and undermines the other individual. At worst, this is bullying. It is embarrassing to admit but anyone who works in any healthcare system has experienced this in some form. There is no excuse for it. It leads to tears, resentment and formal complaints.

There is a more persuasive reason to encourage radiologists to be more affable, aside from being a better person and not getting sanctioned. It is simply that civility saves lives. It isn't that incivility directly kills patients. It is just that incivility is part of a recipe for poor medical care. There is now overwhelming evidence that if someone is rude to someone else, a whole web of unpleasantness unfolds.

The main effects are on the recipient of the uncivil behaviour. They take it personally, becoming stressed and anxious. They lose time worrying about the rudeness, they reduce their commitment to work, they avoid the offender, reduce their time at work, reduce the quality of work and take it out on patients.

But also the witnesses of the uncivil behaviour are affected, both other staff and patients too. The performance of those nearby also suffers and they become less willing to help others. Patients feel more anxious and less enthusiastic for those giving care to them.

So, as you can see, not being rude isn't about being loved and avoiding trouble, it is about good medical practice. Faced with such overwhelming argument, I hope you will agree that a quick and easy temper is clearly a sign of an inferior and uncultured radiologist. Whereas a steadfast and unflinching radiologist is part of the solution for modern healthcare.

And this is where equanimity comes in. This is a concept worthy of exploring and adopting as your default option in times of stress.

In 1889, Sir William Osler's famous address 'Aequanamitas' captured the *zeit-geist* of the late Victorian era. A medical man at that time (and they were virtually all men) was supposed to be a sober and upright citizen, in complete physical and mental control. It was a philosophy of life encapsulated in a single word, from the Latin for 'with even mind'. Coolness and presence of mind in all circumstances was seen as the premier quality of a doctor.

In Osler's day, physical control or imperturbability was important to ensure clear judgement and to maintain the patient's confidence. One didn't want to appear flustered or panicked. Given that medical practice in those days largely concerned the rather inexact science of clinical diagnosis and the even less exact science of prognosis, maintaining the confidence of one's patient was paramount. Confidence was important back then. Losing the patient's confidence often meant your services weren't retained and you didn't get paid.

Mental control, or equanimity, was seen as equally vital to physical control. Calmness and inscrutability allowed clearness of judgement in moments of grave peril. This attribute was nurtured in young doctors and medical students through encouraging patience and persistence. In full development, such as that seen in an older colleague, it was seen as akin to a divine gift, a blessing and a comfort to all who came in contact with them.

Of course medical practice at the time was very different to today. Whilst great strides were being made in the understanding of disease, the investigative arts were basic—pathology was king and radiology didn't exist yet, although Röntgen's famous discovery followed 6 years later.

This said, there are still similarities to Osler's time despite the technical sophistication of modern medical practice. Life is still uncertain, truth is still fragmentary and the demands of successful medical practice are still challenging. But a number of false assumptions have arisen about equanimity. Equanimity has become a negative and outdated concept. This implies an imperturbable doctor is emotionally constipated, hierarchal, haughty, uncaring and inhumane. The spectre of a white male authority figure is raised, complete with frock coat and alarming facial hair.

A few things. I should stress that Osler didn't want his young colleagues to deliberately fake this emotional state. He didn't want them to construct an artificial emotional barrier to hide behind. He stressed heavily that imperturbability is derived from wide experience and an intimate knowledge of disease. Such expertise affords protection against circumstances that would normally disturb the mental equilibrium.

This resonates with me. A deep knowledge of the conditions I am scanning for allows me an inner calmness. I am on familiar turf. I've seen it all before. Even when something unusual crops up, I can handle it safely and calmly. But it is difficult to mask the sense of unease when I'm out of my depth, on unfamiliar ground and struggling to make meaning of an unfamiliar scan.

Osler then expounds on how this isn't the same as hardness of demeanour. An uncaring attitude was a criticism of the medical profession even then. Osler only advises 'insensibility' or immunity to emotion when 'steadiness of hand and coolness of nerve' is needed. He advised cultivating a cheerful calmness and that doctors meet the trials of practice with courage and 'a smile, and with the head held erect'.

Again, this makes sense. You don't want to bottle it half way through a procedure just because a smidge of 'house red' (i.e. blood) gets sprayed up the walls. You don't want to burst into tears in front of a patient just because you see liver metastases on the ultrasound. You don't want to be unable to complete a report because you are so upset about the greyscale tragedy unfolding on the screen in front of you. Acknowledge the emotion but you must press on and finish the task.

One of Osler's little observed points is a misquote from Shakespeares *Antony and Cleopatra*, 'from our desolation only does the better life begin'. Life inevitably contains disappointment, perhaps failure. You cannot avoid such matters. But he advises that by standing up bravely against the worst and, irrespective of victory or defeat, emerging cheerful is the making of a wise, peaceable and gentle doctor. And who wouldn't want that?

Chapter 4
Rule #4 / / Work Hard

It is the radiological trump card, "Yes he may be a sociopath with BO that makes paint peel but he works hard." But don't work too hard. You only have a finite time on this planet.

———

Not long ago I organised a teaching day for our local radiology registrars on 'Becoming a Consultant'. Looking for a job after 5 years of radiology training can be a matter of considerable anxiety. This anxiety is misplaced. Consultant radiologist vacancies across the UK are widespread and unlikely to change anytime soon. It is widely acknowledged that if you have the FRCR exam, a spine, a pulse and at least one good eye, you are in. And most employers are not that fussed about the spine to be quite honest, although no invertebrates have applied just yet.

Anyway, we'd dragged the great and good from around the region to say a few short words. Being a bright-eyed bunch, the assembled acolytes listened assiduously to the advice of the assembled authorities.

One particularly sparky colleague started his talk by asking the audience, "How long does a consultant interview last?". There was brief muttering and murmuring before sporadic replies of "thirty minutes", "forty-five minutes" and "one hour" came back. After a short dramatic pause, he smiled knowingly and answered, "five years; it has already started".

Suitability as a future consultant radiologist is judged throughout training. As the majority of radiology trainees end up working in the region where they trained, it is important to nurture a good reputation from day one.

If a radiologist wants to be popular with non-radiologists then they cultivate what is known as the 'Three As'. These are (in order): 'Availability', 'Affability' and 'Ability'. Being immediately accessible is number one by some margin. The importance of having a radiologist on tap is something that clinicians, clerical staff and others want first and foremost. Next, they want someone pleasant. They want a radiologist who will not just listen and be reasonable but be welcoming,

P. McCoubrie, *The Rules of Radiology*, https://doi.org/10.1007/978-3-030-65229-6_4

charming and easily biddable. Technical ability takes a firm back seat. It is perhaps assumed but is not the primary motivator.

Radiologists judge each other quite differently. They primarily rate each other on their ability to get through work. Of course this isn't unusual in a profession; many others around the world are judged similarly. But radiology is unique amongst the medical sub-specialities in the emphasis it places on volume of work per unit time.

The reason for this is fairly simple. The workflow of the radiologist reporting a scan comes near the very end of a long scan pathway. If they don't do their job, the turnaround time from request to report suffers. If the department doesn't get the scans turned around quickly, it has several effects. First, patients might well suffer through the delay. Probably no harm is done by the odd day here and there but weeks to months is a different issue. Second, you get a bad reputation when, in fact, everything else may be A1 perfect. Thirdly, it creates more work. You start to get a trickle of notes, emails and phone calls asking for scan results. This then builds to a veritable river which then strangles your ability to work efficiently.

Not only do you need radiologists who'll shift the work but they also needs to be both reliabile and flexible. Thirty scans per half day is phenomenal, particularly if you do this day in, day out. But thirty one day and none the next is no use. Plus if you dogmatically insist on thirty scans, irrespective of the work needing to be done then you are a bloody nuisance.

Perceptions of inflexibility and unreliability provokes resentment. Even if the perception isn't real or just exaggerated it still affects the team dynamic. Given repeated offences, the team starts to falls apart and the work suffers. The best radiology departments are full of reliable yet flexible workhorses who get the work done with the minimum of fuss. The worst radiology departments are full of prima donnas whose inflexibility is only outstripped by their piss-poor work ethic.

Of course, radiologists spend less than half their time actually reporting scans. In some workflow studies, they spend around 40–50% of their working week actually sitting at a PACS station. The rest of the week, we attend multi-disciplinary team meetings and clinico-radiological meetings, we vet and protocol scans, we teach others and we do procedural work. But, curiously, reporting workload is seen as core and the rest as a mere side show.

The pre-eminence of a work ethic amongst radiologists is given such priority that it seems to be over and above such niceties as personal hygiene, appearance and professional behaviour. I've worked with some radiologists that look (and smell) like a tramp. But, by jingo, if they bulldoze through the work, all is forgiven. I've worked with some radiologists that are cantankerous and sullen. But incivility is tolerated if they demolish work like a cartoon Tasmanian devil.

Work ethic is a peculiar notion that we all bandy about without further thought. The word 'ethic' implies it is all optional, a path we choose or a personal belief. There is also a moral tone. Those with a good work ethic are Good; those without are Bad.

To a certain extent this isn't particularly unfair. Good work ethic involves arriving promptly, settling down the job in hand without prevarication and working solidly within minimal breaks until the working day is done. Working hard entails churning out more work per unit time than is the average. And we radiologists are definitely judged on such productivity measures. There are whole systems of work that have been developed to judge this, such as Radiology Value Units and the Korner system.

The problem is that work ethic is quite different to above average productivity. It doesn't bear critical examination at all. In fact, confusing high productivity with a good work ethic starts to create problems. It starts to create biases that can be quite destructive. I'll explain.

Demanding high productivity isn't fair to younger radiologists. A radiologist at the beginning of their consultant career is roughly half as productive as a radiologist at the end of their career. Surgeons and other doctors in the 'craft specialities' physically slow down with age. They may be wiser and more experienced but they are less productive. Not so with diagnostic radiologists. Over the age of 55, they are worth their weight in gold. It is therefore common for young radiologists to feel undue pressure about their productivity. They feel obliged to work well in excess of their paid hours to combat their inexperience. Whereas older radiologists can have an appalling work ethic, be an awful colleague and yet be relatively highly productive.

There is a further major flaw of overly promoting number of reports per unit time as a goal in itself. You inadvertently encourage people to play the system. There are many ways that this can happen, some deliberate and cynical, some subtle and often done subconsciously.

Obviously the quicker you work, the better your reporting numbers look. So it makes sense to seek out work that is quicker to report. I won't steal the thunder of Rule #73, but suffice it to say that cherry picking the easy work is most unwelcome in a radiology department; it is inexcusable, like flatulence in a small reporting room.

An inevitable aspect of working too quickly is that quality suffers. This is a variable feast. A common scenario is an overworked radiologist, trying desperately to finish the days work and by working a little faster than normal, they make minor errors. But at the other end is what has been called the 'potted plant' radiologist who barely glances at the images.

A 'potted plant' as a radiologist would be, from a work output point of view, ideal (Fig. 4.1). Show it a radiograph and the lack of reaction can be taken as the plant thinking this is normal. In fact, you can show the plant many hundreds of studies an hour and the reaction will be the same. And given that over 95% of radiological studies are normal or near normal, it's error rate will be <5%. And who wouldn't settle for an accuracy rate of >95%? I've met a few potted plants in my time. When I was young, I used to be in awe of their work rate. Now I can't watch them; it is like nails down a blackboard.

Many fine words have been written about work:life balance. Like many others, radiologists fight against the constant ingress of work into their unpaid and precious home life. Some are very good at rigidly protecting their own time, others less so. There is a curious pleasure from being a workaholic. If you enjoy

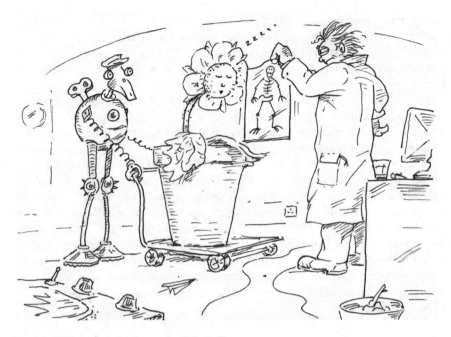

Fig. 4.1 "The 'potted plant' type of radiologist"

your work and are good at it, such passion can be source of considerable reward. It enriches your life with meaning and purpose rather than causing misery and burnout.

However, most radiologists don't get many kicks from progressively working harder and harder. They want less *curriculum* and more *vitae*. And only the individual radiologist can decide on this balance. All I'll say is that you'd struggle to find a radiologist who had 'I wish I'd spend more time at work' on their gravestone.

Chapter 5
Rule #5 / / Toughen Up

Modern medical practice is tough. Patients still die despite all best efforts. Other doctors aren't always nice to each other. No one said it would be easy. Develop a thick hide, become stoical and just get on with it.

—

When people talk of resilience in medicine, I reach for my metaphorical revolver. I cannot abide this. Of course doctors have been dealing with emotional and potentially upsetting subject matters for millennia. And there is evidence that you can teach people how to be better at it. That isn't why I get upset. The thing that annoys me is they are usually shifting blame away from the institution and onto the individual.

Institutional resilience simply must be differentiated from personal resilience. They are quite different topics. Institutions, such as hospitals and their radiology departments, need to cope with anything that might be thrown at them. Institutions are reliant on adequacy of planning and resources. They must have sufficient capacity, sufficient redundancy, and sufficient contingencies.

Whereas we humans only have our mental resources to call on. We have finite capacity and limited mental redundancy. We can and should have contingencies. We can and should have resources to be able to call upon. But increasingly individuals are being blamed for institutional failures.

This simply isn't on. Victim-blaming ruins lives. First that of the staff, they suffer as victim then accused. Then, as a knock on, the patient suffers. In certain countries scapegoating of medical staff is rife. I have been told that it is beginning to affect public transport as so many doctors are being thrown under a bus.

You would have thought we live in a more enlightened age. Sadly, all evidence points to the contrary. Health institutions at a local, regional and national level do not act in a mature fashion. Mainly as there are far too many politicians involved in health. I can't speak for every country in the world but as a rule of thumb, most

© The Author(s), under exclusive license to Springer Nature Switzerland AG 2021
P. McCoubrie, *The Rules of Radiology*, https://doi.org/10.1007/978-3-030-65229-6_5

health systems are resource constrained. And resource-poor systems revert to type, they overload the individuals because of lack of institutional resources.

Now this isn't every institution. The airline industry, for example, has adopted a Human Factors model. They explicitly look at what went wrong rather than who was wrong. But if the plane is on fire before you take off, it doesn't fly. If the pilot or other staff are on fire, the plane doesn't fly. If the passengers are on fire, the plane doesn't fly. Medical practice continues irrespective of who is on fire. And, just to clarify, when I say 'on fire', I mean this as a metaphor. Hospitals and the people in them should not literally be on fire. Nope. Never.

You'll note I am speaking generally about hospitals and medical practice. And you may be wondering quite how radiologists fit into this. You'll also note that I am speaking quite vaguely about resilience as a concept. You might even say, "Ha! Radiologists have it easy, they don't need to be resilient".

To a certain extent, you are right (see Rule #76). Particularly diagnostic radiologists. The most common dilemmas that I face day-to-day in the workplace are the precise number of espresso shots and the choice of bean. But the bedrock of procedural radiology is different. The standard radiology 'list' (i.e. half day of back-to-back procedures) will entail meeting a rapid succession of people for the first time, doing something brief but unpleasant to them, then leaving.

Most patients are fairly stoical. They accept that the radiologist has a job to do and it is nothing personal. Obviously the degree of procedural unpleasantness varies. At the benign end of the spectrum is ultrasound. Although an ultrasound scan is a benign procedure, one should never underestimate the unpleasant shock of cold coupling jelly. Particularly when it is liberally applied to the nether regions. The degree of risk is usually proportionate to unpleasantness. There is very little harm that you can do with an ultrasound machine. Apart from, perhaps, when thrown violently from close range.

At the other end of the spectrum are a massive array of minimally invasive techniques that make up the canon of interventional radiology. Few modern radiological procedures are so unpleasant as to need a general anaesthetic. The days of, say, translumbar aortography are, thankfully, long behind us. But these aren't benign procedures. The more life-saving a procedure is, the more risk there is of something going drastically wrong. The stakes are high in particular parts of the body. Footling around in the small arteries of the brain with catheters is not too far removed from chainsaw juggling. One false move and someone loses the use of a limb. Or worse.

I've witnessed deaths as a radiologist. But to be honest, I had no hand in the causation of them. Nor did any of the other staff. It just happened that the individual randomly ended their life in the radiology department. This is a statistical issue. If over 1000 patients a day visit your department then a health event will occur eventually. Most are minor but some will be serious. We deal with them as they arise. They can be upsetting but no one feels guilt over these; they are just random bad luck.

Sometimes the causation is indirect. Every radiological procedure puts stress on the patient's body. If you are in poor health and if the stress is prolonged then things can go wrong. Something simple like straining on the porcelain throne afterwards can be enough to trigger a cardiac event. Most often this is just self-limiting vasovagal faint. But it can be a fatal event. Although Elvis is said to have glamourised this way to meet one's maker, I can confirm that expiring on a hospital toilet is the antithesis of an attractive end.

Sometimes you are involved in a last ditch attempt; the patient is dying and you are attempting to stop them doing so. Quite often such attempts are forlorn, irrespective of your skill. If you fail, it is easy to rationalise such failure as nature taking its course. You remember the instances, of course. They can be very traumatic. But the lack of causation is a balm that assuages guilt.

Rarely, a radiologist will accidentally cause harm via their own actions. A complication will occur, the procedure will fail and the individual will suffer. At mildest, the patient suffers bruising or a mild allergy. Sometimes, at worst, death.

Although I'll talk more about complications in Rule #32, iatrogenic complications are the bane of a radiologist's life. Needless to say, it takes a certain amount of mental steel to cope with a patient dying on the end of your catheter. Of course, your suffering is nothing compared to that of the patient and their family. It is one of many reasons that I don't do interventional radiology—I am a complete chicken. Plus I have 10 thumbs for fingers.

But it isn't just procedural radiology either. The world of diagnostic radiology has its stressors in equal but different measure. The main stressor, if I'm quite honest, is overwork. It's an old joke but diagnostic radiologists are like mushrooms; we are kept in the dark and constantly have crap piled on us. The stress actually comes when you are constantly interrupted. Or you being asked to do an impossible amount in a short time. Often this comes whilst trying to work in an unsuitable environment, without the right tools for the job. Most of us can cope with this but if it is persistent it can lead to burnout.

The two main others stressors in the life of a diagnostic radiologist are errors and unpleasant colleagues. Again, I will deal with errors in Rules #50, #51, #77 and unpleasant colleagues in Rules #8, #30, #38, #43.

But cope with the rough patches we must. The key is not to bury them, suppress them and forget about them. It is tempting to think that it might be protective to deny that you have flaws or are in some way imperfect. But this isn't about you and your ego. Egos and radiology are a dangerous mix. Ignore your hurt pride and potential tarnishes on your reputation. Coping constructively with hard times at work is about being able to function properly at the very least. At best, you can use adversity to grow wiser and stronger.

This is the crux of this Rule. To toughen up is to grow as a professional despite the slings and arrows of outrageous fortune. By cultivating personal resilience a radiologist doesn't let failure or difficulty drain their resolve. They get knocked down and bounce straight up again. Except they bounce up slightly stronger than before.

How can you do this? Well, it doesn't come easily but it can be developed. First step is culturing an unwavering cheerfulness as we discussed in Rule #2. This is a pre-requisite. The second step is to develop control of your emotions, as we discussed in Rule #3. Again, this is not an option. The next step is to examine the situation for positive learning points. Then, whilst acknowledging and accepting the negative feelings, make an adjustment and get straight back to work. The last step is to look after yourself. But you'll have to wait until Rule #99 to read more about that.

Chapter 6
Rule #6 / / Respect The Machines

Don't verbally abuse the scanner or let it know you are in a hurry. They have sensors for that and will shut down. They are particularly sensitive after 4.50 pm, Friday afternoons, on the birthdays of loved ones and on anniversaries.

—

Radiology is now almost 100% technology dependent. We cannot function without an array of electronic devices. The days of X-ray films on light boxes are long gone. Certainly this is true in the UK; we went 100% digital in 2006. Others around the globe have done likewise.

For reasons that escape and infuriate me, films and light boxes still make widespread appearances on TV medical dramas. Possibly that the production team have a ready supply in the props room and it makes a set look more hospital-y. Whatever the reality, a modern medical drama always has a light box in the background. And the chest x-ray on said light box is either upside down or back to front. Or, more usually, both. It is an old tradition, a charter or something.

Not only have films gone but everything else in radiology is digital too. Dictaphones and their tapes are a thing of the past. Secretaries rarely do any typing these days, voice recognition software has seen them off. Although we still issue paper reports, they'll be gone before too long.

This digital revolution means that if there is a power cut, we are hamstrung. The whole digital system can grind to a halt very easily as the delicate daisy chain of electronic co-dependencies needs to be working slickly. You'll note I specifically said 'working' and 'slickly'; just 'working' isn't enough.

This digital edifice is known as PACS. A point of principle here. PACS stands for 'Picture Archiving And Communication System' but some radiologists waggishly comment it might as well stand for 'Pain And Constant Suffering'. A minor point to raise is that 'PACS system' is incorrect; it is a tautology like 'skin rash'. Using this phrase marks you out as amateurish and ill-informed. PACS is just

P. McCoubrie, *The Rules of Radiology*, https://doi.org/10.1007/978-3-030-65229-6_6

PACS. I know that I'm being pedantic again. But if pedantry annoys you then this is not the book for you. There is much much more to come.

At its most basic, PACS is just a computer network which allows (i) image data to be sent from scanners to storage servers and (ii) computer workstations to retrieve data from the servers so as to look at the images. There is, of course, more to it than that. But radiologists know how the rest works and others would be bored by a deeper explanation, so I'll skip the techie stuff.

Of all the different machines that are key to the work of a radiologist, the scanners come first and foremost. You can't do anything unless there is an image to work from. And when I say 'scanner', I'm talking about any radiology kit that produces medical images. At the low end, bog-standard x-ray machines and at the top end space-age, bells-and-whistles scanners like PET/MRI.

Oh, and another thing. We radiologists don't talk of an 'MRI scan' or a 'CT scan'. The word 'scan' is another tautology. Just CT or MRI says everything. Plus, if you want to sound like a radiologist, you must abbreviate MRI to MR. This is, of course, pronounced 'em-aar' not 'mister'. You'd get some strange looks if you go to the scanner and announce that you'd like to organise a "Mister Brain".

You also hear of 'CAT scans' but this is a double no–no. Computerised axial tomography was it's original name in 1971 but hasn't been called that for decades. You are only allowed to use this phrase if you are over 90 years old or attempting a weak animal pun, usually involving 'PET scans' too.

Scanners demand respect as they are astonishing bits of engineering. When Arthur C Clarke started his third law, 'Any sufficiently advanced technology is indistinguishable from magic', I always imagine that he was envisioning the latest scanners. For example, when a CT scanner spins a 2 tonne gantry at 180 rpm, it rips 28G and yet you can balance a coin on top when it is going full tilt. The latest MRI scanner is 7 times the strength of a scrapyard electromagnet, cooled to $-269\,°C$ $(-414\,°F)$ by liquid helium and contains a 10 kW radio transmitter. Not far off magic.

Ironically, older scanners are often more reliable. They are less complex and their foibles are easily worked out. Radiology departments also tend to keep the reliable scanners and ditch the newer and more troublesome ones. Some scanners that were like a bike I had for years. It was the same bike apart from I'd changed the wheels, frame, seat, brakes and entire drive chain. Only the handlebars were the same.

One of our old CTs was like that. It had the original shell casing but everything else had been replaced, often several times. I remember when the ball bearings on the gantry gave out and it came to an abrupt crunching halt. The engineer later found out it had spun over 2 million times before this terminal event.

Scanners also deserve the care and respect that you would show to a temperamental colleague. Modern scanners are hardy as the moving parts are durable but anything that moves will eventually break. The scanner software is like any software—mostly fine but prone to irrational and unpredictable freezes. I'm not saying the scanners are sentient. You'll never find emotion detectors specified in the technical blurb. But the pattern of breakdown is uncanny. Always just when you least want it. The machines must have some way of detecting the most inconvenient time to blow a gasket.

There is no good time for a scanner to breakdown. Plus the NHS is not exactly over-provided with scanners. So any down time is bad news for a department. But it seems that the more you rush, the slower the scanner goes. The more emotion-laden the scan outcome, the more likely it is to freeze. The more tension in the scanner control room, the more it glitches.

Experienced staff know this. They exude calm as their fingers dance over the control knobs and buttons of the scanner. This deliberate calmness pervades the atmosphere. The invisible sensors don't go off and the scanner functions as normal. This is why experienced and calm staff are absolutely vital when dealing with urgent scans. Elbow the newbies out of the way; let the grey-haired ones drive the machine.

PACS similarly plays up at the most inopportune times. Radiologists view PACS with love and hate in equal measure. A latter day radiological ying and yang, if you would.When PACS works slickly, radiologists can motor through the work. Far from impeding progress PACS can positively boost productivity. When PACS is playing up, it can turn the calmest and most saintly radiologist into a snarling purple-faced monster. The frustration can boil to the point of technological defenestration. It is probably a good thing that radiology reporting rooms don't have windows—the temptation might be too much.

The optimal approach to PACS is to adopt a zen-like attitude from the outset. Sit down and before switching it on, focus on inner peace. Then boot it up and remain emotionless as it loads up. If it then works adequately, be happy and tranquil. When it inevitable slows, crashes or stops working (and given enough time, it will) then stay calm then turn it off and on again. There is no point in expending even a microjoule of emotional energy. Not a single shouted word, gritted tooth or thumped table will improve its electronic behaviour.

Getting upset with computers is like getting upset because your train is running late—both are exasperating but almost entirely out of your control: you are essentially powerless. Thou shalt chill thy beans. The difference between rail transport and PACS is that if the train stops, you can't exactly turn a train off and on again, enjoying a cup of coffee whilst it restarts.

These enforced coffee breaks are no bad thing in themselves. Doctors are notorious for poor eating and drinking habits. Most beverages are sipped at a workstation and the keyboard forms an expensive plate for sandwich crumbs. The odd enforced break here and there isn't a problem but recurrent or prolonged breaks due to PACS downtime can become a real issue.

Hence an enforced break from work isn't enjoyable if you don't want one. No one likes being powerless over their work pattern. It is also doubly frustrating as during any PACS downtime, the scanners keep churning on. The longer PACS is down, the more catching up there is to do. And radiologists are busy enough, thanks very much.

Thankfully, most PACS vendors have cottoned onto reliability as a number one issue. And they occasionally listen to radiologists so that their products aren't so bloody unusable. But the real ire of a modern radiologist isn't now aimed at PACS. It is aimed at voice recognition (VR). But you'll have to wait for Rule #86 to find out why.

Chapter 7
Rule #7 / / Never Let A Clinician Play Radiologist

If the request gives specific radiological directions, you must do the opposite. A request for 'CT with contrast' means they get an unenhanced scan; any request for "obliques" gets just an AP and lateral.

—

Some time ago I published this Rule in an official publication of an esteemed UK radiological institution. Modesty prevents me naming the specifics. Well, modesty and a vague concern of legal action. Anyway, my words attracted a sternly-phrased letter to the editor.

The rather po-faced author, who shall also remain nameless, took this rule at face value. Mistaking my humorous intent for a literal instruction, they admonished me at length. We are talking proper shroud-waving with a bit of hellfire and brimstone thrown in. The letter finished with the intention to give me a sound spanking. Actually, I may have made up the last bit. But you get the gist. Needless to say, the editor and I shared a brief giggle and filed it 'in the big round file' (i.e. binned it).

There will always be mirthless types in radiology. You know, the tight-lipped sort who can't tell an olecranon process from a thrombosed haemorrhoid. The ones that wear white socks with black shoes. You know. What that mirthless individual didn't understand is that this Rule is simply poking fun at a perennial issue in radiology. This issue is where a clinician starts telling a radiologist how to do their job. Any radiologists reading this will smile in recognition. They've been there and seen this. Every day. Usually several times a day.

I should probably clarify the word 'clinician' as I use it with specific intent. It means someone who works predominantly in the clinical arena; a ward, a consulting room, an operating theatre, that kind of thing. It is someone who is patient-facing for the majority of their working day. No longer does it mean exclusively another doctor and hasn't done for decades; plenty of other professional groups have a case load and hence ask for scans. I'm not that keen on the phrase 'Allied

Health Professionals' but there is no better name for senior nurses, physician associates, senior physiotherapists and so forth.

Obviously some radiologists can have quite substantial clinical roles and do work in such areas, particularly the modern model of interventional radiology, with clinics and dedicated day-case units. But 'clinician' denotes someone who asks for scans as part of their overall clinical responsibility for the patient's care. This differentiates from the clerical staff who also ask for scans but their role is to cajole, to expedite and coordinate.

Anyway, back to the Rule. You might think I'm being a terrible stick-in-the-mud. Surely the clinician is just trying to help you do the right thing, aren't they? Well, I'm sure they think they are. The issue is that they are wrong 95% of the time. And the other 5% of the time, their instructions are superfluous. I realise that this is a bold assertion but stay with me, I will explain.

So why do clinicians overstep this line in the sand so frequently? I think that the majority of it is ignorance and only a small part is arrogance. They have no idea of the professional boundaries that they are trampling all over. Of course clinicians naturally want the best for their patients and they assume, wrongly, that more is better. More views, more contrast, more specific directions. Just more of everything. Occasionally they think they know best—after all, how hard can this radiology lark be? This is tired yet familiar story of a little knowledge being a dangerous thing. I'll give some examples.

(1) *Specifying Views.* We have a local knee, erm, 'specialist' who always asks for 4 specific views on all knee X-rays, irrespective of the clinical problem. In the Big Book of Knee X-rays there are several different sorts you can do. But 99.99% of knee X-ray examinations are just two views—one taken from the front (AP) and one from the side (lateral). It seems that this specialist thinks that adding the words 'Skyline & Rosenthal' to their requests makes them look cleverer.

Whereas, being honest, additional views rarely add anything. Or rather there is a law of diminishing returns. The third view adds only a little; the fourth less still and further views are almost useless. Anyone asking for (or performing) six views as a routine needs a long hard look in the mirror. If I was braver I'd tell them to sod off; they can have two views like everyone else. I'm minded to avoid the obvious and real excuses such as radiation protection and resource limitations. I might try fobbing them off with 'sorry, we've run out of X-rays'; fending off idiocy with counter-idiocy.

(2) *Specifying Contrast Media.* There is also an allegorical surgeon who 'orders' each CT abdomen with 'everything', specifying oral, intravenous and rectal contrast media. The more contrast, the better the scan, right? Except it doesn't work that way. More contrast rarely helps. Contrast isn't risk-free and occasionally it paradoxically makes scans harder to interpret. The rule here simple; leave the contrast decisions to the radiologists.

The biggest problem with contrast is that most normal people don't enjoy being given it. Moreover, of all the orifices into which one can instil contrast medium, rectal has to be the second least favourite (after urethral). And the oral stuff tastes nasty; gratuitously unpleasant. The very existence of Gastrografin is an affront to patient-centred radiology. Of all the contrast media in all the countries in all the world, my hospital still uses this stuff. Come the revolution, when I have the reins of power, I'm banning the stuff.

(3)   *Gratuitous Instructions.* This is another common peccadillo. For example I get requests asking "please scan the abdomen and please comment on the liver". What exactly did they think I was going to do? Ignore the largest organ on the scan? Wilfully omit any mention of the 1.5 kg lump of flesh in the right upper quadrant? When I read this nonsense I can't help wonder if the same people write referral letters to others saying 'Thanks for seeing Mrs Bloggs for further assessment. Oh, and don't forget to take a medical history and perform a physical examination too'. I'm sure they don't mean to be patronising but they are.

(4)   *Post-processing demands.* A more modern infraction goes beyond witless suggestions of technique. It intrudes very much into the dark heart of radiology. This type of referral makes specific demands in the post-processing of the images. It'll say something like "CT Head with coronal recons". What the clinician fails to realise is that all data from a CT scanner is post-processed. The raw data from the scanner is fed into a very powerful computer that constructs a stack of data, best visualised as a very detailed Lego model. Where the individual lego pieces are sub-millimetre cubes.

Once this stack of visual information has been produced, reconstruction is just a few mouse clicks away. Radiologists have been reconstructing images in the coronal, sagittal and any other plane they want for over a decade now. This image processing and reformatting is just part of what radiologists do to make better sense of the image. Just occasionally we'll prepare some images for surgeons to help plan their operations. But that is it. The point is that post-processing is 95% for the radiologist. It isn't for anyone else. So any external post-processing imperatives just serve to rankle.

Given all these irritating intrusions, it is quite easy to see how a radiologist may become peevish. They make take this rule literally. My advice is to rise above this. I encourage my clinical colleagues to submit 'blank forms' when they aren't sure what precise test is best. I say to them 'tell me what the clinical problem is and I'll do the right sort of scan for you'. This approach generally works well.

I should stress that this Rule isn't about protectionism or turf wars. That is a completely different topic altogether. Other healthcare professionals have long been performing scans and procedures that were traditionally performed by a radiologist. It'd be pointless and unnecessarily antagonistic to moan about this.

I'm also ducking the issue because turf wars are dull. Anything partisan tends to be acrimonious for those involved and tedious for on-lookers. This book aims to edify, enlighten, enthuse and amuse. With turf wars, you just can't do any of that. There is nothing big or clever about petulance and squabbling. There are a few decent jokes that I could make. Sadly they would offend everyone who isn't a radiologist.

The only thing I will say is that I have no problem working with anyone who is fully trained, who works as part of a team and works cooperatively to help maintain and develop a quality service. Untrained or part-trained individuals doing their own thing without any integration into the bigger picture are a positive menace. You wouldn't have it in any other industry or branch of medicine. We shouldn't tolerate it. End of.

Chapter 8
Rule #8 / / Forgive The Sins Of The Clinician

They are just jealous. There are two types of doctors: radiologists, and those who wish they were radiologists. After all, we have the most expensive toys and the comfiest chairs.

—

In Rule #7 I clarified the distinction between clinician and radiologist, highlighting one of the more common sins of the clinician. The interface between radiologist and clinician is obviously important given how central radiology is to modern medical practice. The interface has both a front end and a back end. The front end is where the request is received and the back end is where the results are communicated back to the clinician.

The receiving and issuing ends are the two aspects of a radiology service that clinicians see. Obviously this is completely different to the patient's experience. But it is worthwhile considering what happens after a radiology request is received, mainly to illustrate the many points of potential failure that can occur.

If you consider this journey from request to report, this pathway through the radiology department, you begin understand the beating heart of radiology. If you map out the processes and pathways of a radiology department, you'd unearth a colossal spider's web of actions and interactions. A fair-sized department like the one I work in sees around 1500 radiological examinations a day. At any time there are literally thousands of these studies snaking their way through the system.

Most of this is hidden from view, kept quite deliberately back of house. Clinicians and patients don't encounter the minor horde of clerical staff who are specifically employed to manage this. Every radiology department manages each of these journeys on a particular specific bit of software called a RIS or Radiology Information System. This links to several other hospital systems, including PACS. It usually links to an electronic system of requesting studies, clustered under the loathsome name of 'ordercomms'.

All departments in a hospital and surrounding community will have their own unique computerised systems that need to connect to everyone else's systems. Consider this and you begin to see why healthcare IT has a notoriously bad reputation. Integrating these systems should be simple but the reality is, as ever, a story of singular frustration. You might that that having one big computer program that looks after every bit of the hospital would work better. The problem with a one-size-fits-all approach to IT is that one-size-fits-no-one.

Such is the complexity of modern radiology that it is a minor wonder that it works at all. I point out these back-of-house processes as any can be meddled with by people outside the radiology department. Believe you me clinicians can and will interfere with these, often unthinkingly. The litany of sins of the clinician is almost endless.

This Rule is fairly simple. It is about rising above moaning about one's clinical colleagues and the day to day annoyances they inflict upon us. It asks radiologists to adopt of an attitude of pitying forgiveness. We should forgive them because, well, that is what civilised humans do. As Jesus had it, 'Forgive them; for they know not what they do.'

A radiologist should pity clinicians. I should clarify what I mean here. I use 'pity' quite deliberately. You may read this and think 'you smug git' and, to a certain extent, you'd be right. But not in that way. I'm not using 'pity' in a contemptuous fashion. I don't mean a sneering superiority kind of pity. Don't be condescending towards clinicians. It achieves little apart from winding them up and making you look like a jerk.

It is also useless if you are pitying but just sit and watch dispassionately. This can be construed as insulting, if you think about it. You have recognised a problem but you have not taken action. The implication is that you have judged it unworthy of your action. Pity can be a virtue only if you then act with compassion. When we help our sinful clinical colleagues, one should do this full of kindness.

Clinicians are definitely jealous of radiologists. Some are open and frank. Some will grudgingly admit it. The rest would never say it but they are. It isn't that being a radiologist is generally excellent (it is—see Rule #74) but more that being a clinician is so unutterably awful these days. It seems that, in the last twenty years, all the things that made it worthwhile being a physician, a surgeon, a general practitioner or whatever have either eroded or gone completely. The clinical arena seems, to my admittedly jaundiced eye, to be a cesspool. A shark-infested cesspool.

As a result, in the UK, radiology has never been so popular amongst medical graduates. Currently, there is a four to one ratio of applicants to places, the highest of all the mainstream hospital specialities. I can't speak for other countries but I don't hear of unemployed radiologists or unfilled training posts.

This jealousy takes many forms. They are jealous of many aspects of our work and our working conditions. Often the clinician will voice explicit gratitude after a mutually rewarding case discussion. A civilised confab can be a salve for a stressed soul.

Jealousy from clinicians is often tacit. It isn't unusual for a clinician to look at a radiological image and whistle softly in astonishment, murmuring phrases of wonder. Sometimes it is entirely non-verbal. I'll paint you a common picture of day-to-day life where I work.

We have, like many places, dedicated reporting rooms. I am lucky as I work in a recently built hospital. The reporting rooms are air-conditioned and dark. The only noise is the hum of the computers and soft swearing of a radiologist, cursing the Voice Recognition system (see Rule #86). Not all radiologists are so lucky. The first fifteen years of my radiological career were spent working in pretty antediluvian conditions. I didn't know it at the time. It is clear only in retrospect.

Anyway, enter the consultant surgeon (Fig. 8.1). She wants to look at a scan and has tracked you down. She struts into our dimly-lit workspace, fresh from the melee of clinical practice, all bustle and activity, steam metaphorically arising from the ears. She exhales into the four-point adjustable chair next to you and her eyes widen briefly at the contrasting serenity. As she takes in the comfort of the chair, she osmoses the tranquility. Within 15 seconds, the head slumps back onto the headrest, the shoulders unwind, the eyes close momentarily and they sigh wearily. Some surgeons get so comfy that they kick off their shoes and curl up slightly. I've stopped short of offering a blanket and mug of cocoa.

Not all clinicians are so pleasant about it. Their jealousy spills over as resentment. They are slightly bitter about the contrasts between our mutual work and working conditions. Rather than be congratulatory or even aspiration towards us, they seek to ruin our working practices. You may think this far-fetched but, whilst uncommon, I've experienced it first hand.

You have to remember medics can be extremely competitive. A minority of medics want to win at all costs. Because they cannot make their practice any more enjoyable by fair means they aren't averse to negative tactics. They cannot have others be happier or more successful than them and so drag everyone else down to their level. They do this by denigrating radiology and radiologists. They paint radiology as an irrelevance, quite peripheral to medical practice. They dismiss radiology as easy-peasy, something they can do easily. Individual radiologists are painted as over-privileged; precious, soft-handed, work-shy fops. They falsely paint the cost of scanners as an outrage, pooh-poohing the need for new or replacement scanners as a radiological vanity project.

You may be reading this and feel disbelief and a sense of outrage. Do radiologists honestly come under assaults like this? It isn't common but yes, we do. I'm not pretending others don't nor that we are particularly hard-done by. Every trade, every speciality has their own menu of annoyances to chose from. But faced with these pernicious barbed comments, it is easy to see why radiologists can hold substantial grudges.

Who doesn't hold grudges? I'm still annoyed by things that happened decades ago, some perpetrated by people now long dead. But grudges aren't anything to be proud of. They are a dysfunctional badge of anger, a open psychological wound, part of a victim identity. They don't work either. Grudges make you bitter,

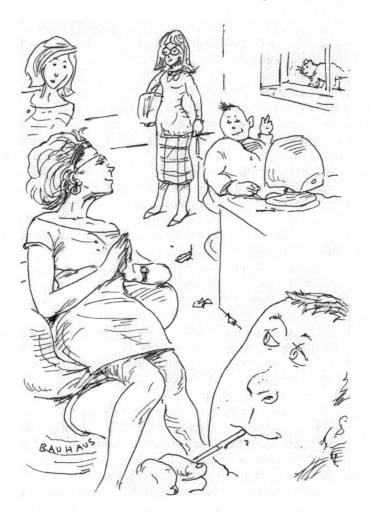

Fig. 8.1 "Enter the consultant surgeon"

depressed and anhedonic. They lead to intolerance and incivility. Intolerance leads to a silo mentality and a whole host of jingoistic nonsense.

The opposite of a grudge is forgiveness. Forgiveness is a marker of personal enlightenment and a thing to aspire towards. It isn't easy to turn the other cheek, to soak up abuse and still carry on. The keys to forgiveness are dispassionate attention towards the underlying causes (see Rule #38), acknowledgement, acceptance, and focussing attention on positives. If you move through those stages, you can forgive and let it all go.

Forgiveness isn't easy. I really struggle with it. But the worthwhile things in life rarely come easily. Attaining radiological nirvana takes time and effort. It takes a single-minded effort to become consistently compassionate. But you must. Positive collaboration and cooperation with clinicians is the only way to get good health outcomes. And it is for this reason that radiologists must forgive the sins of the clinician.

Chapter 9
Rule #9 / / Don't Be Too Approachable

You don't want to be the one who gets asked to do everything anymore than you want to be the one that everyone slags off as being grumpy and lazy.

—

One of our trainees, who was duty registrar at the time, said to me just recently, "I can't get any proper work done for all these interruptions". I smiled. It is true. Radiologists view interruptions as a pox on their working life. But I smiled as it also revealed an unconscious bias so blatant that it might as well have been tattooed on their forehead: their concept of 'proper work' is producing radiology reports.

Reporting activity is all these days; it is the über-metric. Gone are the days when the worth of a radiologist was their sound opinions, the eloquence and lucidity of their reports, their humanistic qualities, their abilities as a teacher, researcher and all-round good egg. If you ain't shifting a thousand studies a month, then you ain't worth nuffin'. At least that is how it feels, even if your boss denies it emphatically.

Anything that impedes reporting is, therefore, an annoying distraction. Tensions do rise when you can't seem to get any 'proper work' done. After the *n*th individual physician has swung by your PACS station that morning you can hear a vague swooshing sound as your reporting target whistles past.

There is no doubt that it is annoying to have your intellectual reverie shattered. The typical interruption comes midway through the oncology case with monthly pan-body investograms spanning a seven-year history with sixteen separate index lesions.

Only two types of interruption are welcome. The first is the appearance of a colleague wanting to chew the proverbial fat for five minutes. Not only is this usually a welcome break but can be seen as much-valued in-house Continuing Professional Development. The second type of interruption comes after an a few hours of wading through seemingly endless plain radiographs. You've been using

© The Author(s), under exclusive license to Springer Nature Switzerland AG 2021
P. McCoubrie, *The Rules of Radiology*, https://doi.org/10.1007/978-3-030-65229-6_9

basal ganglia alone and even they are protesting. The prospect of re-engaging the neocortex via human conversation is often appreciated.

A knock on the door or polite cough is the usual announcement. The more senior and, well, *surgical*, the noisier the arrival. We have a local neurosurgeon who has been known to announce their presence in the form of song, I kid you not. However, some folk sidle in completely soundlessly and you only become aware of their presence by some bizarre sixth sense.

The interloper typically opens with "Can I ask you a question?". I have tried the answer "And your second question is?" but most blink momentarily at this repartee, before launching into their prepared spiel. The other classic of "Can you vet this scan?" can be countered with "I'm a radiologist, not a vet". Witty as I think this may seem, no one has ever laughed with 100% honesty at that one either. Their expressions are usually that of bewildered pity.

The task that is asked is usually inversely related to the time you have available. Most mornings will only see trivial queries about, say, bunion-ograms, Whereas at 4.55 p.m. on Friday, the patient is always someone very young, very complex and very sick. On the birthdays of spouses or beloved offspring, all hell tends to break loose bang-on quitting time whereupon you find yourself mysteriously without a single colleague in the entire department.

A variable length of time later the trespasser has departed, your cup of tea has gone from lukewarm to stone cold and your mental radiology cache has auto-deleted. You sigh audibly, mentally ruminate about the precise dates of your next booked annual leave, and then turn back to the tombstone-like PACS monitors to start afresh.

And yet despite all this bellyaching, it is a radiologist's job to be interrupted. Well, not quite. It is a radiologist's job to be consulted. It is all in title. We in the UK and much of the Commonwealth call our senior hospital doctors 'consultants' and have done for many decades.

This is opposed to an North American 'attending' who, presumably, does a little more than the title suggests. 'Attending' sounds a little passive, if you ask me. It is almost like they don't take their coat off and just watch through the glass. But it seems to work for our cousins across the pond so I'm happy for them.

In many ways, an experienced radiologist on the front line in a problem-solving role is a highly effective model. Radiologists are used to making quick decisions based on minimal information. It is what we do all day, every day. Furthermore, radiologists like to be in control of their workload (see Rule #67) and are keen on making sure the department works slickly. So, it works.

Except it doesn't. There are many reasons why it doesn't work.

- First, radiologists are quite an expensive asset. If you want someone to do reception duties; you hire a receptionist.
- Second, the better service you offer, the busier it gets. Along the lines of 'build it and they will come', if folk know they can get instant access to a senior radiologist, they'll grab it with both hands.

- Third, any consultant-led system needs enough folk on some kind of rota that doesn't fall apart at the hint of annual leave. Organising a radiologists's rota is like passing a kidney stone; extremely painful and with no guarantee of success.
- Fourth, it is ironically more difficult to arrange in larger departments due to increasing specialisation. It would be nonsensical, for example, for the most senior interventional neuroradiologist to be asked to speak to a general practitioner about a toe X-ray.
- Fifth, at least two duty people are needed. You need a front-of-house radiologist hot-reporting plain radiographs, fielding the calls, vetting and protocolling. Being interrupted during a plain film is no problem. The second rostered radiologist is the looking at the complex inpatient and emergency CT and MRI. They second radiologist needs peace and quiet.
- Last, front door consultations obey a law of diminishing returns. A small effort helps a lot but bigger effort only helps a little more. As we seem live in perpetual straitened times, generous staffing of the front end of the radiology department with senior radiologists is a luxury that most cannot afford.

The real trick is to try to differentiate unnecessary interruptions from consultations. The former doesn't need a radiologist, the latter does. To be honest, you rarely know which it is going to be when the door opens or when the phone rings. And the door of a reporting room bangs like a barn door in a hurricane and the phone chirrups like a crazed canary.

There are many ways to distinguish interruptions from consultations. Each radiology department does it slightly differently, evolving organically. For example, my old radiology department had a 'Ron'. Ron had worked in the department for decades in a variety of roles. He knew everything and everyone. He was endlessly calm and knew how to cajole even the most prickly personalities. He was the single point of contact and revelled in helping folks out. He was known and loved across the hospital for capably handling any query. Of course we didn't know what we had until he retired. And boy did we miss him when he went.

A single Ron is fine for a small to medium size department but not for a large department. It is just too complex and busy for one person. You need a combination of systems. What doesn't work is unsmiling faces saying "no", locked doors and unanswered telephones.

A triage system is necessary, where non-medical staff filter out as many queries as possible. They then sign-post to the most appropriate radiologist. Once you remove these unnecessary interruptions, then you can start calling them consultations. Once you see them like this and you see them as an important aspect of clinical practice, you start bringing the value-added nature of a clinician-radiologist discussion to each case.

Senior clinical colleagues want rapid access to specific radiologists. Make them jump through hoops and they resent it—their time is equally valued. Lock the door and they'll kick it down. But this access shouldn't rely solely on goodwill, it should be planned deliberately. This is critical. For example, if timetabled, you can plan for it. A classic example is regular morning meetings. In many groups (trauma, neurosurgery) this is established daily practice. Some are a bit behind the curve. But such meetings have a massive benefit. For example, daily meetings between abdominal surgeons and abdominal radiologists change patient management in 30% of cases.

But not every query is planned or coincides with the 0800 daily meeting. Not every question can be handled by the duty radiologist. As so, irrespective of any triage system, radiologists will get a regular number of phone calls, queries and consultations.

This is where it helps to be a 'Goldilocks radiologist'. In the fairy tale, Goldilocks wants porridge that is neither too hot nor too cold, she wants a bed that is neither too hard nor too soft and so forth. A radiologist that is grumpy, lazy and unreliable will be loathed and shunned. Whereas a radiologist that is lovely, alway says yes and alway delivers will drown under the weight of work. A Goldilocks radiologist treads the fine line between the two: they keep clinicians happy yet have a manageable workload.

Chapter 10
Rule #10 / / Be A Good Colleague

A good radiology department is one where you show cases to each other on a daily basis. Experienced colleagues get their egos checked; younger colleagues get a helping hand. If you aren't doing this, you might be part of the problem.

—

I read a question on social media recently that read, "What three best things at work make your professional life feel warm, happy and satisfying?". I thought about this for at least a few microseconds before answering "Colleagues, colleagues and... colleagues".

It is a truism that with good colleagues you can pretty much cope with anything. The support and camaraderie are everything. And, lets face it, being a radiologist in today's NHS isn't a walk in the park. We've got work coming out of our ears and are expected to work in relatively wretched surroundings. I'll explain.

A few years ago I had occasion to visit all the radiology departments in our region. What floored me was how damned shabby they were. Most people don't notice this squalor—it is normal for them. I was acutely aware of it as our new hospital had only just opened and the difference was quite stark.

In the hospitals I visited, the radiology reception and patient waiting areas had been smartened up in various ways but the back-of-house areas had usually not seen a lick of paint in over twenty years. The furniture was misshapen and ramshackle. Things were held together with tape. There were odd holes in floors and walls. And to be quite frank, some departments smelled a bit funny.

I don't think it was the staff that smelled. Your average radiology department worker is typically the hygienic sort. Working in small dark rooms for most of the day makes you quite aware of such matters. The smell I am talking about is a peculiar institutional staleness. It is an ingrained and slightly sour odour that has accumulated over decades. It isn't from lack of cleaning. But it can only be solved by ripping everything out and starting afresh.

© The Author(s), under exclusive license to Springer Nature Switzerland AG 2021
P. McCoubrie, *The Rules of Radiology*, https://doi.org/10.1007/978-3-030-65229-6_10

A colleague recently came up with a beautiful mixed metaphor, saying, "He was so busy, he didn't know which fire to piss on". The UK currently has one of the lowest number of radiologists per capita in Europe. It's a shambolic 20+ year-long tale of piss-poor planning. Yet demand keeps rising. The UK's Royal College of Radiologists has estimated a 30% increase in workload in the last 5 years.

It is on this backdrop that most NHS radiologists work. You may think I'm plucking the strings of the sympathy violin a little hard. But I'm not after pity. I'm merely painting a picture, setting the scene. It is a hostile environment. So you need all the help you can get so as to cope with it. This starts with having good colleagues. A good colleague can take many forms but there are five key elements for a radiologist.

These are (in order):

(1)   they are a safe pair of radiological hands; this is a *sine qua non*;
(2)   they work hard (see Rule #4);
(3)   they are pleasant to everyone (see Rules #2 & 3);
(4)   they are flexible;
(5)   they readily discuss cases with you.

Whilst the last one is specific to radiology, the first four aren't rocket science. You could say the same sort of thing in any trade or medical speciality. But it does need pointing out. Mainly as these things need to be borne in mind when recruiting. And also when negotiating with a difficult colleague. These are, after all, The Rules.

To a certain extent you are stuck with the colleagues you have at the time you are appointed. But they chose you and you chose them. You have to work on the presumption that they thought you'd be a good fit. I see nurturing close relationships with your colleagues as very important. I'm not talking about living in each other's pockets or holding parties that entail swapping of spouses. Just spending a little quality time each day catching up. Plus, if they ask for a favour, always do it if you can.

There is a point behind this, other than being a decent human being. This is the concept of 'Investing in the Bank of Goodwill'. This notional repository is key to good relations with your colleagues. If you do a favour for a colleague, you are making a deposit. A big favour is a big deposit. You need to build up your account because you never know when you'll have to ask a favour in return. And you also don't know how big a withdrawal you're going to have to make.

It is very reassuring to know your account is well in the black. But if you neglect your account or if you go overdrawn, you'll find colleagues strangely offish and reticent to help. Go badly overdrawn and you'll find support lacking when you need it most. Ask for help and colleagues will turn their backs.

Recruitment of a new consultant is a big deal. Consultant radiologists tend to be monogamous, usually staying for over 25 years in a single hospital. So it is important to get it right. There is an adage that you should chose your colleagues more carefully than your spouse as, over the years, you end up spending more time with your colleagues than you do with your spouse.

Appointing medical staff is a bit like shopping for clothes according to doctor and novelist Colin Douglas. He explained in a BMJ Column that interviewing a fellow consultant is like buying a new suit. The result has to last, so you spend maybe 40 minutes. Appointing registrars is more like buying a shirt. No sensible panel would give it than 15 minutes. And more junior doctors? "Nobody wastes a lot of their time buying socks".

Selection is not an exact science. The svelte bright new hope can turn out to be disappointingly narcissistic and avaricious. The ugly grey duckling that you appoint hoping for a glorious swan can fail to blossom, staying grey, stolid and unexciting. You appoint in hope, looking at potential. What happens in the first 5 years of their consultant career is, in part, up to them but also on how they are treated by their colleagues.

Time and energy invested in a new consultant radiologist by their colleagues is normally a sound investment. If you see the new kid on the block as someone to dump all unwanted duties on, you'll engender resentment. Whereas if you are supportive, non-judgemental and kind, you'll bring out the best in your new colleague.

What I am describing is mentoring. This is simple and uncontroversial. It isn't specific to radiology or even medicine. It is embarrassing I have to point it out. But success is mainly about doing the simple things every time (see Rule #82). It is quite accepted in many professional circles, even senior practitioners can benefit. But sadly such practises are far from routine amongst NHS consultants.

I don't know why it is not more commonplace. Maybe it is some misplaced notion that a consultant should be fully trained and needn't ask for help. Perhaps having help from a senior colleague is seen as a sign of weakness. But this is codswallop. Absolutely everyone in the trade knows that the learning curve as a new consultant is particularly steep. It takes at least 5 years to get your feet under the desk. I have no idea why we don't formally support our newer colleagues as a routine.

Psychotherapists and counsellors will be very familiar with 'clinical supervision'. This is where practitioners of all vintages have regular meetings to discuss their workload. It is a step away from mentoring but not far off. Many other groups have cottoned on to this way of working. Nurses and all manner of health professionals are doing it. But not doctors. Nope. Rare as hen's teeth.

But until some form of mandatory enlightenment is forced on doctors, the best single step individual radiologists can take is showing cases to each other. By 'cases' I mean something specific. This is all the relevant radiological studies together with available clinical history pertaining to a particular 'health episode'. Non-medics think it odd to thing of ill people as 'cases' but it is a just a way of coldly analysing the facts, just like a detective working a case.

There are several reasons why showing each other your cases is a great way to develop and maintain expertise.

– First, it is natural and informal. There is no stigma. It is a Good Thing. No one can or will object to it.

- Second, it fits easily into the working day. A colleague swinging by to show a difficult or interesting case is a welcome distraction.
- Third, it taps into the hard-won knowledge and experience of your colleagues, mainlining pure expertise for free.
- Fourth, the mental processes of experienced colleagues are deconstructed and laid bare. Complexity is easy to assimilate when broken into bite-sized pieces.
- Fifth, there is emotional buy-in. If it is your case or that of a close colleague, it is more meaningful and hence more memorable.
- Last, it is uniquely interactive, quite unlike a lecture or journal article.

I hope you now agree that colleagues of all ages should show cases to each other on a daily basis.

Chapter 11
Rule #11 / / Never Measure Anything

A radiologist with a ruler is a radiologist in trouble. If you can't measure it with the eyeball-ometer, you are out of your depth. Accurate measurements honestly don't matter. The nearest centimetre or so is absolutely fine.

—

I read a radiology report a while ago that contained this little beauty, "The right kidney measures approximately 11.27 cm". It is a wonderful example of a poor sentence. It reads plausibly but those six words strongly signal something deeply amiss. You will have spotted the major clanger of using 'approximately' with a precise figure. But there are more subtle issues which I will unpick for your reading pleasure.

Unless you have wielded an ultrasound probe in anger, you might not know that most ultrasound machines measure to two decimal places by default. A colleague used one that states distance to three decimal places. To be honest, I wouldn't be surprised if someone somewhere is writing a radiology report that includes measurements to nearest angstrom unit.

This is why software engineers shouldn't be given too much rope. I'm amazed at the profusion of ineptly designed bits of software in radiology. Clearly the majority have never been wafted under the nose of a radiologist. There is one bit of famous software that was written by a radiologist (Osirix). I remember using it for the first time was epiphanic. It was like stepping into a warm jacuzzi after having walked half a mile barefoot on a Lego road.

Anyway, back to the measurement. You may be thinking to yourself that there is nothing wrong with high levels of accuracy in our measurements. The main issues are that highly accurate measurements are (i) impossible to perform reliably, (ii) not actually necessary in the majority of cases, and (iii) often unnecessarily and crudely reductionist.

I'll explain. Since Röntgen took his first image in 1895, people have been keen to improve their ability to assess radiological images. There are endless studies

© The Author(s), under exclusive license to Springer Nature Switzerland AG 2021
P. McCoubrie, *The Rules of Radiology*, https://doi.org/10.1007/978-3-030-65229-6_11

looking how accurate they are at doing so. Specifically, researchers want to know how reliably different people are at measuring or assessing the same things. This is known as inter-rater reliability. It is a bit of a Big Thing in radiology. Essentially, unless a specific technique or measurement has this in spades, it never catches on.

Obviously it depends on what you are measuring and what you are using. Measuring fog with a bit of string is quite different to measuring a ball bearing with a micrometer. But if, for example, you measure the aorta with ultrasound, you should be able to get to correct figure ±3 mm. Given that an aorta should be less than 3 cm it means that repeated measurements by different operators should be accurate to within 10%.

Note the aorta is usually a uniform tubular structure with sharp margins. Good images are easy to obtain. Most things that radiologists attempt to measure are irregular and ill-defined. Images aren't always perfect either. So real life measurements are much less accurate. The lesson from this is that give or take 10% is about as good as we can expect. Highly accurate radiological measurement is a tautology. Precision is a myth.

This isn't a flaw or fault. It is just the simple limit of human accuracy with a specific tool. You might think that computerised measurement must be more accurate? I could write a whole tedious chapter on why this isn't true. Just take it from me, computers aren't there yet. They'll get better. But in the meanwhile, take any automated or semi-automated measurement with a hefty pinch of salt.

This give or take 10% rule works well in practice in virtually every radiological modality. It is also a handy hint when monitoring something. And we monitor a lot of things these days. Sometimes it is for good reasons, sometimes for dubious reasons, sometimes for absolutely no reason whatsoever. But irrespective of the intrinsic worth of your measurements, a good radiologist looks for trends over time, ignoring minor variations as background noise.

Different cancers grow at different rates. You may be aware of 'volume doubling time'—the time a tumour takes to double in volume. This is a long-standing way of judging how aggressive it is. They can be thought of as either tortoises, hares or birds.

For example I was looking at a scan of a kidney tumour recently and I calculated it's volume doubling time to be 1100 days. After watching it for nine years, it had finally struggled to one inch in diameter. This is a 'tortoise', an indolent and non-aggressive thing. It can be left alone.

Many cancers are 'hares'. With a volume doubling time of, say, 100 days, they are sprightly beasts that need hacking out pronto. Some cancers, like some lymphomas, are like 'birds'. With doubling times in the order of 15 days, you don't have time to monitor them, they rear up and fly away before your very eyes.

The 10% rule and volume doubling times don't really work so well for small things. In fact, no approach works well for sub-centimetre lumps. Measuring to the nearest few mm is difficult to do reliably. With the one exception of kidney stones on CT, the majority of small things are a nightmare for radiologists.

At 3 mm or less, you are going to struggle to even see the blasted thing. It is just too small. And even if you see it, you can be pretty much sure it'll turn out to be nothing. In fact, there is an argument that lumps <3 mm are virtually always benign, that if you mention them you are doing the patient a disservice. Most radiologists specifically ignore most tiny incidental lumps for these very good reasons.

Pure maths dictate that you are in trouble around 4–10 mm. These lumps are small and hence difficult to perceive. Again, the incidence of trouble is very low. Depending on the organ in question, up to 95% of these lumps are benign incidental findings, often called 'incidental-omas'.

You are doubly in trouble as volume is the cube of diameter. A 4 mm lump is difficult to pick from a 6 mm lump. But a 6 mm lump is nearly four times the volume. And a 10 mm nodule is twice the volume of an 8 mm nodule.

Like I said, measuring <10 mm lumps is a fraught business. Judging change on serial scans is horribly inaccurate. It is why volumetric techniques and semi-automatic lump analysis isn't a mature and useful technology just yet. And I daresay it might never be terribly useful.

But let us consider the 'eyeball-ometer' for larger lumps. Experienced radiologists know what I mean. After measuring the same sort of thing 5000 times, you get fairly slick. You can estimate the size of something quite accurately and extremely rapidly with the unaided eye. You certainly don't need a ruler.

I have a maxim of 'the nearest centimetre or so is fine'. Some people have taken extreme exception to this maxim. I'll explain why it isn't controversial. It isn't that I don't measure things. I do. But I measure to confirm what I've already eyeballed and decided on. In fact, I measure as the last step after I've looked hard at all studies, looking in all 3 planes. I certainly don't measure first and decide later.

This maxim is a rejection of slavish adherence to unthinking measurements. Measuring everything doesn't make you a better radiologist. In fact, stating measurements is largely useless as the vast majority of your target audience have no idea what these figures signify.

This maxim is questioning traditional measurements. We routinely measure the length of kidneys. We routinely measure the cardiothoracic ratio on chest radiography. But these measurements, like most others, are pretty bloomin' useless. The eyeball-ometer of an experienced radiologist is far better.

This maxim is also a rejection of arbitrary size classification. There are plenty of classification scheme in widespread radiological use that have strict size cut-offs (i.e. RECIST, TNM). They directly cause a tsunami of radiological measurements. Generation of these is laborious and is of diminishing returns. In fact, most radiologists who have had anything to do with RECIST get heart-sink at the sight of those six letters.

Most experienced radiologists distrust arbitrary classifications. Classification schemes arise when a panel of grey-suited, grey men decree that, for example, a 2.1 cm breast cancer is profoundly much worse than 1.9 cm tumour. Clearly this makes no sense. It might be a bit worse but 2 mm is neither here nor there. Such thresholds are clearly arbitrary.

Douglas Adams famously wrote that the answer to life, the universe and everything was 42. It is an enduring and brilliant joke as it the perfect *reductio ad absurdum* argument. To summarise all of human existence as a number is utterly, utterly absurd.

It is also absurd if radiology reports are dominated by numerical measurements and classification systems. I'm not railing against measurements or classification systems. Far from it. But they should have their place. A radiologist that churns out reports that are primarily a list of numbers and figures is doing it wrong. The narrative, the nuance, and the humanity gets lost amid the jargon. And such reports are fundamentally unreadable, which is never good.

Hence a good radiologist describes the appearances first and foremost, makes the minimum of pertinent measurements as a secondary action and applies any classification system as a low-key finale.

Chapter 12
Rule #12 / / Never Count Anything

If you are trying to equate quality or experience with activity, you are missing the point. You could be doing the wrong thing over and over again. Anyone who brays about their 'numbers' is indeed an ass. If counting is the sole rationale, you are the wrong person to be doing it.

—

Robert McNamara, US Secretary of Defence 1961–8, was famed for quantification. Previously a successful businessman, he was renowned for decision-making on numerical observations. Under his direction the Pentagon modelled military success in Vietnam with the traditional metrics of victory. Key information, such as total enemy dead, was gathered by Army Intelligence (a beautiful oxymoron, if ever I saw one).

This was nothing new. But McNamara ramped up the authority and scope of this process. If it could not be measured, it was not important. But there was more. Personal insights were ignored. External data were ignored. Questions about the data were ignored. Fundamentally the war didn't yield to numerical analysis. This led to a monumental failure of strategy. The Vietnam war lasted 19 years, cost billions and killed millions.

Sociologist Daniel Yankelovich introduced 'The McNamara fallacy' in 1972:

"The first step is to measure whatever can easily be measured. This is OK as far as it goes.

The second step is to disregard that which can't be easily measured or to give it an arbitrary quantitative value. This is artificial and misleading.

The third step is to presume that what can't be measured easily really isn't important. This is blindness.

The fourth step is to say that what can't be easily measured really doesn't exist. This is suicide."

© The Author(s), under exclusive license to Springer Nature Switzerland AG 2021
P. McCoubrie, *The Rules of Radiology*, https://doi.org/10.1007/978-3-030-65229-6_12

The parallels to radiology are immediate. Radiology lends itself to a metric-based approach because each X-ray, scan or procedure is easily counted. 'Patient episodes' or 'attendances' are the quanta of radiology. Data can be generated with a few mouse clicks; workload is quickly tallied. A logistical hop, skip and a jump later and *voila*—you have targets.

Radiology can be heavily target-driven. Targets are obviously intended to promote good practice and they can work well. I remember in the early 2000s before targets when our waiting time for routine spinal MRI was 2 years. With enforced targets this dropped to 2 weeks.

But targets really do show the full glory of the McNamara fallacy. The immediate problem is that targets become de facto measures of quality. Complexity and subtlety is sidelined. Unquantifiable attributes such as compassion and caring count for nothing. This is madness. It indicates you've truly lost your way. You might think I'm posturing but witness the UK's Stafford Hospital scandal.

Measuring radiology workload is simple but measuring quality is complex. Unfortunately target culture is so ingrained that our higher and betters firmly believe that complexity can be tamed by further analysis. If there residual doubt, collect more data. This leads to a labyrinthine infrastructure of data coding, gathering, refinement and analysis. This spits out stacks of stats that singularly fail to clarify what good looks like.

Now this is ok if the stats are easy to gather. Invalid but not harmful. But it would be wholly inappropriate for radiologists to become, in essence, very expensive data inputters. We are the wrong people to be counting things.

This situation is even worse when data has to be gathered for external inspection. This is no way to improve quality. If you 'pass', you've wasted your time. If you 'fail', it is too late. Plus there is the aggravation and grief as well as the time and energy wasted by you and them. External inspections waste £millions every year.

Another problem is encapsulated by Goodhart's Law. Named after the British economist Charles Goodhart, it can be paraphrased as 'When an outcome becomes a measure, it ceases to be a good measure'. This acknowledges the unintended behavioural consequences of target culture. Most often this is simple gaming to improve such metrics without any regard for improving quality. Occasionally it forces a dumbing down, stripping away complexity and subtlety purely to service the metric. But it can lead to grotesque outcomes, some occasionally harmful, all at odds with their original intentions.

There are many unintended consequences of target culture in radiology. I could write a whole book on them. But I'll illustrate with a few of my favourite motifs:

First is the widespread tactic of setting a new demanding target. Crucially both stick and carrot are at play. The carrot is short-term transitional funding. The stick is a monetary punishment if you fail to comply. The intention is that short term funding will result in a lasting improvement. But it rarely works. The end result is doing more work for the same money. Which translates to existing staff having to work harder.

The second notion is raising professional standards to improve quality. This is unarguable—our patients deserve the highest quality care. The result is a tightening of control on training and accreditation. This is now the premiere method to solve all healthcare ills. UK medical practice is probably the most highly regulated in the world.

Except this doesn't work. Our health outcomes are no better than other countries with less regulation. This isn't the whole story though. This 'tightening control thus protecting patients' motif is used as a stick with which to beat us. Health outcomes are not improving so it must be the doctor's fault. Meanwhile, the vast majority of honest and competent doctors will waste time and energy jumping through administrative hoops. An example is UK's Revalidation, costing £100m a year with few proven benefits.

Third is another odious trend. It is the assumption that competency comes with simple repetition. To a degree this works for procedural and interventional radiology. Do it a number of times and you get physically slicker. However, the visuo-perceptive skills of a radiologist are more complex.

Visual expertise is a curious phenomenon. Psychologists are just starting to unpick it. Pattern recognition is an oversimplification; it is way more than that. But expertise does rely on accruing 'film miles'. This ill-explained, non-foveal visual skill derives from years of experience and enables you to spot a lung cancer in 0.01 seconds.

So, yes, experience counts for a lot. But experience must be varied, broad ranging, and of varying difficulty or complexity. It needs reinforcement by feedback, teaching and other learning. Repetition alone is fairly useless as it induces confidence but not necessarily competence. And as we all know, confidence without competence is a route to professional hell and damnation.

Much of radiology training focuses on numbers: numbers of scans reported, numbers of procedures performed. Radiologists know it is an oversimplification but few realise the depth of this fallacy. Such 'educational bean-counting' is easy to administer but fundamentally wrong.

It ignores the breadth, and length, and depth, and height of the experience. Other highly valid sources of learning such case discussion, peer learning, case archives, textbooks, journals, courses, and conferences are disregarded. You could argue these are equally valid and complementary ways of learning.

The unintended consequence is that training becomes a quest to achieve logbook numbers. The totality of experience is short-circuited by this lust for padding out the columns. Less scrupulous trainees guestimate their numbers with varying degrees of overestimation. Whereas the assiduous trainees waste hours meticulously recording everything rather than actually learning. Pure numbers are therefore not only crude and educationally invalid but easily faked and therefore fairly useless. I think that, overall, logbooks have little role in professional training.

Just occasionally, numerical assumptions are a little more sinister; they are hegemonic assumptions. For those unfamiliar with the term, hegemony refers to the political and economic control exercised by a dominant class. It also refers to the success of the dominant class in projecting its own particular way of seeing the world. The end result is that this is accepted as common sense and seen as part of the natural order by those who are in fact subordinated to it.

Let me illustrate. It is easy to count how many studies a radiologist has reported. These raw figures can be modelled (e.g. Radiology Value Units (RVUs)) to express the productivity of a radiologist per unit time. I don't know of a radiology department that doesn't routinely generate these. Sometimes they as public property—akin to a league-table. In some countries, your productivity is linked to your pay.

The hegemonic assumption is that productivity is the primary method of judging the worth of a radiologist. But it isn't true. Good radiologists can be absolute machines, pumping out reports ten to the dozen. Or they can be plodding and ponderous. I've also seen highly productive radiologists who were god-awful. There is so much more to being a good radiologist than purely churning out masses of reports.

But the agenda of our political masters is different. They want us to work our socks off. Sod the human cost; cost-efficiency is everything. I assert that this is wrong. A civilised society would balk at this notion. Any department with reporting productivity as a primary goal will fail in other respects. Striving to increase reporting productivity is a spiral without end; a death march. Highly productive radiologists feel frustrated and can burnout. Slower radiologists may resort to gaming and other maladaptive behaviours.

Farmers say, "You don't fatten a pig by weighing it". This is as valid for swine as radiologists. Counting things rarely works and is often counter-productive. Be a radiologist that feels the quality not the width.

Chapter 13
Rule #13 / / The Default Is To Say 'Yes'

There are 2 sorts of radiology requests; requests from a competent and knowledge-able colleague, which you accept; requests from an incompetent and bumbling colleague, which you accept right now. Saying 'no' always involves more work in the long run.

——

When I was a fresh-faced consultant my hospital had just one slow CT and one slower MRI scanner. They weren't slow back then but were sluggish by modern standards. Every inpatient scan was discussed to ensure appropriateness. We did about thirty scans a day, total. And that was flat out from 9 to 5. Except, quaintly, the CT scanner closed 12.30–1 p.m. so staff could have a lunch break.

Now we have five zippy CTs and five slightly less zippy MRI scanners. Neither close for lunch. All work 12 hours a day as a minimum, churning through a total of around 300 scans a day. So we've got ten times the workload but not ten times the number of radiologists. Much as we'd like to, we haven't got the time to discuss all the scans. But we do like to discuss urgent inpatient scans.

The more complex the patient, the more I want to discuss it. The more sick the patient, the more I want to discuss it. The more urgently someone wants the scan, the more I want to discuss it. This is primarily so we do the right sort of scan at the right time and answer the clinical question as quickly as possible.

It also makes sure the sickest patients get priority. You might think this obvious but clinicians are only human. They will do their utmost to get their patients scanned first. Without proper discussion, the priority scans end up being those where the clinicians agitate the most.

This discussion and scan vetting is a minefield. Get it wrong one way and you get howls of complaint from the clinicians, alleging obstruction. Get it wrong the other way and you get howls of complaint from the radiographers that the scanners are rammed. I'll give you a few examples.

P. McCoubrie, *The Rules of Radiology*, https://doi.org/10.1007/978-3-030-65229-6_13

Imagine the scene. You are the duty radiologist and in strides a clinical colleague. You know them well. You trust their clinical instincts and their judgement. After brief pleasantries and a soupçon of light-hearted banter, they ask for a scan. The clinical scenario is briefly but clearly laid out. You agree that the scan will clearly help that patient. Smiles all round. Further pleasantries, cursory banter, *exeunt.*

Imagine another scene. You are the duty radiologist and in shuffles an unknown person. The stethoscope indicates they might be a doctor. They ask for a scan. You smile and ask politely why they want it. There is hesitation, humming and hah-ing. After fifteen seconds (see Rule #43) the smiling facade has slipped, attention has wandered and fingers are drumming. You ask for a brief summary and alarm bells start to ring in your head. The patient is probably very poorly. You agree to the scan and arrange the scan urgently.

Two different scenarios, you might think. But it could have been the same patient presented very differently by two different doctors. Ok, the first doctor was a known entity but also was a slick communicator. The second doctor was unknown but bumbling. The second could have had a markedly different outcome if the radiologist had lost patience and told them to tell their story walking.

The major point of this rule is that any radiology request should be judged irrespective of the clinician requesting it and the amount of trust you have in them. You have to try to see past potentially poor communication and petty hierarchies. Your duty, of course, is to the patient. The default response to any enquiry should be, "How can I help [you help your patient]?". It follows that the default to any request for a scan should also be 'yes'.

British radiologists have an additional hurdle in the form of strong radiation protection laws in the shape of Ionising Radiation (Medical Exposure) Regulations 2017 (IRMER17). These laws mandate radiologists to 'justify' any patient exposure to ionising radiation (X-rays or gamma rays). This is sensible, really, even if you are not totally convinced by the linear no-threshold model. But many countries have far less prescriptive laws. Hence radiation dose often features in British clinico-radiological discussions, perhaps more than other parts of the world.

As ultrasound and MRI don't entail potentially harmful ionising radiation they aren't covered by IRMER17. But we like to pretend they are. It is, if I'm honest, about rationing of a scarce resource. It feels reasonable to justify ultrasound and MRI like other scans. If nothing else through a moral duty to both patient and taxpayer.

'Discussing a scan' or scan 'requests' may be quaint ideas to many radiologists around the globe. In some parts of the world, the answer is always 'yes'. In certain countries it is practically unheard of to refuse a scan. If you are paid per scan it makes no sense to refuse (see Rule #58). In this set up, clinicians asking for scans are like postal workers—they just drop off the card without further discussion (see Rule #55). Clinicians 'order' their scans like they would a pizza. It is a one-way communication process.

It isn't always about money. Some countries have a medical culture of providing minimal clinical information and omitting clinical discussion prior to a scan or procedure. If the clinician says, "Jump", the radiologist asks, "How high, how often and for how long?". The notion that a radiologist could have any worthwhile input prior to the scan is not even considered. In such places it is the radiologist's job to, essentially, just shut up and do the scan.

I have heard of British radiologists who emigrate to such countries who then have great difficulty acclimatising to such practices. I have to be honest, it is one of the things that dissuades me from emigrating to warmer and better paid climes. I admit to feeling more comfortable with the British system of doing things. I do feel that discussing urgent scans is time well spent.

This is one particularly rewarding aspect of being a radiologist. I like being 'the doctor's doctor', a valued asset to clinicians. We radiologists are usually good at helping other doctors, particularly in discussion of diagnostic dilemmas. We have a breadth of training: radiology is one of the last 'general' specialities. We have depth too: the Fellowship of the Royal College of Radiologists exam is damned rigorous. We have to know all diseases that affect all body systems, irrespective of age and genders. Furthermore, our training specifically focusses on making rapid decisions based on sparse clinical information. These 'rules of thumb' or clinical heuristics are the lifeblood of professional practice and radiologists have got them in spades.

Individual clinicians tend to have a short-list of radiologists that they will specifically seek out. And, in my experience, they'll be utterly frank about the radiologists that they know and trust. Once you are on the short-list, it is a double-edged sword. You are flattered to be trusted and happy to help contribute towards good patient care. But the phone calls can come at awkward times. Gentlemanly discretion forbids too many details but suffice it to say that phone calls over the years have interrupted several normal physiological processes.

When there is mutual trust a clinician can ask seemingly outrageous things of a radiologist. If a favoured surgeon waltzed in to see me and barked, "dance, black and white picture-box boy" then I would be up and gyrating without a question. It works both ways. I've suggested some fairly bold and occasionally counterintuitive things to my clinical colleagues. And because there is trust they … well, they don't laugh in my face.

A big hospital like mine employs over 400 consultants and a veritable army of junior doctors. Each of the latter changes job every four to twelve months. Much of the time I am speaking to someone that I don't know. This anonymity is a blight of the big institutions. Enduring and positive relations are the blessing of the smaller hospital.

However, it isn't always peace and light in a smaller place. I've known several individuals who are terrible with names. Like me, for one. Most of the time we dysnomia sufferers get away with it but there are always awkward moments. At best you actually might know their name but your mind sporadically goes blank. Commonly you might know their face but can't match it to a name. But worse than this is where you get someone's name wrong but they don't have the heart to correct you. You call them the wrong name. Sometimes for years.

The bottom line is that if a radiology request bears evidence of rational thought then accept it, irrespective of your relationship with the requesting clinician, their seniority or their perceived competence. If there is no evidence of rational thought or if there is positive evidence of disordered thought then you must decline it otherwise you perpetuate poor practice. But saying "No" needs caution and isn't to be done lightly (see Rule #16).

Chapter 14
Rule #14 / / Agitation Is Not An Indication

Lack of planning on their part does not constitute an emergency on yours. Let them get away with it and they don't learn the lesson.

—

When I was a newly qualified doctor, a medical house officer, I was the lowliest member of a 'firm'. Firms are a distant memory now but were the team of doctors working for a specific consultant. There was very little doctoring; I was the continuity guy for inpatients under our team. A sentient invertebrate with a computer log-in could have done 90% of it.

I worked for a slightly dour authoritarian Scottish physician. His clinical method was meticulous but absolute. All his patients were reviewed on twice weekly formal ward rounds. Woe betide me if I hadn't organised everything precisely. If the patient's notes were in slight disarray, this was my fault. "I'm veeery disappointed", he would say, glancing up disapprovingly from under his bushy eyebrows. Thereafter, I carried a box of hole reinforcement stickers in my pocket, to repair torn pages of the notes.

There was one phenomenon that I couldn't work out at the time. We always had one third fewer patients on our firm than anyone else's. This made life infinitely more bearable. The goal of being a house officer at this time was to have as few inpatients as possible. I achieved the magic number of zero inpatients once, for three hours. I had no responsibilities and wandered the hospital, unsure quite what to do with myself.

The only way to get fewer patients under your care was for them to either die or be discharged from hospital. Of course dying was never the goal but did happen sometimes despite best efforts. This system incentivised discharging patients. Obviously you wanted to make your patients better so they could leave hospital happily on the road to recovery.

Turfing them out partially-investigated and under-treated wasn't an option (Fig. 14.1). The hospital I worked in had a 'hand-back' scheme. If a patient was

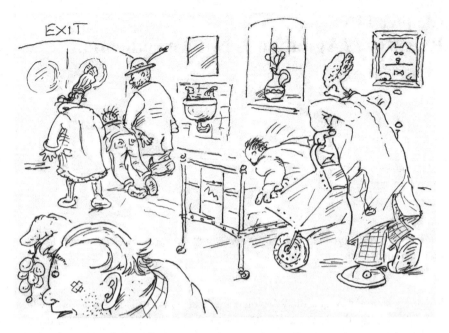

Fig. 14.1   "Turfing patients out"

readmitted that had been previously under your team, they were handed back to you. It was therefore in your best interests to make sure this didn't happen.

I often wondered why our firm had fewer patients. It wasn't that my boss or any of the team had magical powers of healing. We admitted exactly the same sort of patients as everyone else. I only understood this much later, long after I had moved on. It was solely because the boss was exacting. He was highly organised and demanded the same from his team. Our firm ran like clockwork.

This was a hugely valuable lesson. The secret to slick healthcare is not heroics of the individual. Brain and brawn counts for little. It is being organised and methodical. It is working in a system that encourages this through subtle incentives and rewards.

This was reinforced to me during a subsequent job as a medical senior house officer looking after a ward of 30 beds. When one patient died or went home, another patient rapidly appeared. Given this fixed number of patients, there was a perverse disincentive to rapid turnover. In fact, it made sense to fill your beds with little old ladies in no apparent distress (LOLs in NAD—it is a known medical entity). They needed '3 hots and a cot' and next to no medical attention. If they couldn't quite go home yet then that was just fine by me. No one suffered. But patients undoubtedly stayed in hospital longer than was strictly necessary.

As a result of these experiences and many others over the last quarter century, I know what good healthcare looks like: systematic and organised. Accordingly

I'm distinctly intolerant of personal or institutional disorganisation. I am especially intolerant of other people turning their disorganisation into my problem. The Polish have a lovely phrase for this, "Nie mój cyrk, nie moje małpy" which translates to "Not my monkeys, not my circus".

Here is an example for you. So, yes, I understand that the patient has major surgery booked tomorrow morning and they need a pre-operative scan. You are telling me that at 9 p.m. the night before that you want the scan now? And you realise it will need a sub specialist opinion which isn't going to happen by 9 a.m.? I hear that you are most insistent on it, I really do. But it isn't happening tonight.

You may be thinking that this is a ridiculously far-fetched example. Sadly not. You may be thinking that I am a heartless beast. Surely when it is the best interests of the patient, you should get on and do it? Of course, if it is clinically urgent, I would always go the extra mile. But for planned or elective care, it isn't *clinically* urgent. Don't confuse urgency with expediency.

The main issue is having your altruism exploited by someone else's chaotic approach to healthcare. Going the extra mile is a recurrent theme in healthcare. Radiologists do it regularly. We frequently drop everything for an urgent case, staying late or coming in early and a whole lot more. We would happily self-identify as altruistic. And there is nothing wrong with this. It is what we would want for our loved ones should they fall ill.

To this end, altruism is officially encouraged. Removal of self-interest helps focus on the individual patient. Many medical organisations have it as part of their official curriculum, mission statements or whatever. But altruism isn't quite as straightforward as you might think. It is also a hegemonic assumption.

Altruism is fairly simple on the face of it, just describing selfless behaviour for the well-being of another. Understandably it seen as a virtue, a purist goal for all caring professions. It is almost totemic: an unquestionable spiritual characteristic. However, altruism is a hegemonic assumption (see Rule #12) as it actually works in favour of the political overclass.

There are two other big problems with altruism: firstly, although it is painted as being without reward for the individual, this is rarely true; secondly, it's endlessly exploited in the healthcare environment.

Firstly, true altruism entails an absolute lack of reciprocity. There are no rewards for those who act out of pure altruism. But true altruism is rarer than an impoverished orthopaedic surgeon. There are benefits to most supposedly altruistic behaviour if you look. They are subtle, indirect and tacit but very real.

Many apparently altruistic acts have a self-serving element. Consider the act of 'doing a favour'. On the surface, a noble deed. But a favour has a subtext. There is either an expectation of reciprocity or something is done to induce indebtedness. Sometimes the favour is bestowed with a half-hidden notion of improving reputation or social standing. Or an awareness that if the favour isn't bestowed, you could lose face, forcing you do it. When taken to the extreme, this is virtue-signalling; the apparent act of generosity is nothing of the sort. Virtue-signalling is merely a disguised attempt to appear less egotistical.

Second, the bigger issue is the exploitation of altruism. This is rampant in medicine and all the caring professions. Actually it is in slight decline as Generation Y refuses to kowtow to previous norms. But several generations of medics before them (me included) were singularly encouraged to go the extra mile, to stay late, to arrive early, to cover gaps, to soak up more work. It is noble. It is the Done Thing.

Moreover, it is also ingrained. Unpaid extra work is so rife that the NHS would undoubtedly collapse without it. A colleague reckoned that most NHS consultants work an unpaid half-day a week, on average. I agree. I suspect most salaried health workers could tell a similar story of understaffing and overwork.

Here's a few examples of subtle exploitation of altruism:

– You are overjoyed when your hospital buys you a new laptop "to support your on-call work'. This is trumpeted as evidence of investing in their staff. But even if you use it to check work emails at home a few times a month it pays for itself in a year.

– Doctors tend not to go off sick. In fact, it is a badge of honour that you struggle in to work, irrespective of how you feel. This is 'presenteeism'—the opposite of absenteeism. You are at work when you shouldn't be. But you bring infections to patients and colleagues alike. Plus you aren't safe to work—you may actually be a liability. This is exploitative bullshit of the first order.

– A classic is to pretend that a period of extra workload or extended duties is just temporary and things will be better shortly. For example, you work yourself into the ground whilst in training with the promise of an Elysian consultant career. But the cakes and ale never come. The workload never drops. Overwork becomes the new normal.

I've seen all this before and I now reject going the extra mile as routine. I will smile and endure all manner of attempts to persuade me that I should. There are always reasons; someone is always ill, patients are in need of scans. Yes, I know. That is the point of our trade. If someone is properly ill then of course I'll be there. But going the extra mile as a routine is a classic recipe for burnout. As we'll see in Rule #99, a burnout radiologist is a true tragedy.

Chapter 15
Rule #15 / / Always Help The Patient

Helping the medical team is helping the patient. The natural tendency is, of course, to say yes (see Rule #13). Apply the 'grandma test" – what if it was your grandma? Sometimes helping means saying no – it might not be in the patient's best interests (see Rule #16).

———

Many people who've visited a radiology department as a patient will happily tell you their negative experiences. Not everyone; some have a sublime experience and will simply gush about it. Things, however, used to be a whole lot worse as widespread use of non-invasive scanners are a relatively recent feature. A trip to a radiology department would often entail lying on a hard X-ray table looking up at a grim-faced radiologist advancing toward you with a very large needle.

Even now there are various degrees of hardship that are inflicted on patients visiting a radiology departments. Having an X-ray is no big deal, in the grand scheme of things. Having an ultrasound is no particular hardship either. Having radioactive tracers injected is just a fleeting intravenous stab. Ingesting barium isn't too bad but having it inserted anywhere else can be eye-watering.

The contrast media used in CT isn't fun—the intravenous form makes you feel transiently quite peculiar and the oral stuff is unnecessarily vile. Not many actively like going for a ride in the MRI scanner. If you've never had one, the bore of the magnet is alarmingly narrow at around 60 cm (2′) and it is hellishly noisy once it fires up. Unsurprisingly about one in twenty folk bail out before the scan is completed.

I'm constantly amazed by the resilience of some patients. You meet them for the first time and do something unpleasant to them. They then smile and say thank you afterwards. They will endure all manner of invasive and inherently irksome investigations, barely batting an eyelid. We Brits tend towards stoicism. An eyelid flicker may be all we show when a dentist drills a big hole in a bit of gum that escaped the local anaesthetic.

P. McCoubrie, *The Rules of Radiology*, https://doi.org/10.1007/978-3-030-65229-6_15

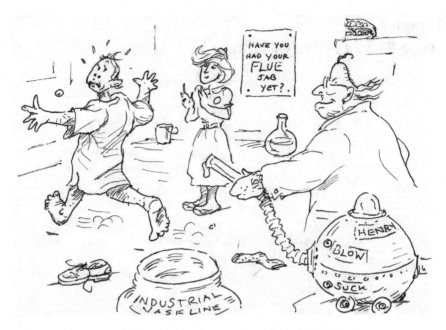

Fig. 15.1   Approach some with a lubricated enema tube and they bolt for the door

Of course not all patients are so stoical. Merely unsheathing a tiny 25 g needle (0.5 mm in diameter) causes some to faint clean away. Approach some with a lubricated enema tube and they bolt for the door before you have time to say 'floccinaucinihilipilification' (Fig. 15.1). Some tend towards the dramatic; wailing and flailing in a manner that can be surprising if you weren't expecting it.

Most patients agree to tests in the belief that the end justifies the means. It is often subconscious. They balance short-term inconvenience with what they see as long term benefits. Specifically it is about perception of pain, risk and inconvenience versus the accuracy and worth of the investigation.

There is also the issue of trust too. Blind faith or 'the doctor knows best' is ebbing away as people seek to be more involved and engaged with their care. I have found that if a patient has faith in their clinician then they will usually agree readily to investigations. Such is the trust that they freely sign up to invasive, risky or unpleasant tests. The doctor-patient relationship is therefore critical when a clinician sends their patient for a scan.

However the harsh reality is that the requesting clinician often relies on blind faith. The conversation with the patient is generally one-way and terse, along the lines of, "I'm going to send you for a test". They don't have the time to explore the patient's beliefs or if the patient wants the test. Many clinicians have little idea of what the test entails either, even if the patient were to ask. The clinician assumes a linear process will occur: the request will be entertained, the scan will be organised, the patient will present themselves appropriately, successfully endure it and the radiologist will generate a report thereafter.

In my experience, the requesting clinician will virtually always overestimate what the patient will happily endure. Some of this is that the average patient these days is older. Older people tend to have more wrong with them and tend to be frail. Hence older people's tolerance of investigations is lower.

The other erroneous assumption is underestimating what the scan entails and any risks to the patient. This is, in part, as they've never had one of these tests themselves. I'm a healthy middle-aged chap but the few scans I've had were no walk in the park. I am in absolutely no rush to have an intra-articular injection ever again.

Put this together and there is a frequent disconnect between the goals of investigation and what can be reasonably achieved. It is relatively common to have a clinician that wants a test to answer their question and a patient who isn't keen to have a specific test. And the person in the middle is the radiologist. We are regularly asked to make decisions about how to achieve the best possible diagnostic outcome with the minimum of patient discomfort or harm.

This is a trade-off. Highly accurate tests tend to be more of an ordeal. Whereas tests that are more acceptable tend not to be terrible accurate. You need a sensible radiologist who knows the foibles of various tests. They then match these to the individual patient and their individual needs. This way the patient can to achieve a diagnostic result without being overtly tortured.

Let me give you an example, a patient with an unexpected iron deficiency anaemia. It would normally be prudent to perform a 'top and tail'—upper and lower gastrointestinal endoscopy to look for a source of presumed blood loss. Colonoscopy becomes riskier and more difficult in the elderly and so we locally offer a CT of the colon to those between seventy-five and eighty-five. We find that those over eighty-five generally don't tolerate CT of the colon—it is quite an ordeal. So we offer the over eighty-fives a CT with just oral prep to fill up the bowel with contrast. Ranking by age is crude and we do tailor it; these aren't fixed, just rough rules of thumb that work well in practice.

Of course the final arbiter of what is right for the individual patient is the individual patient. We constantly ask patients how they want to proceed. Although it seems that there is a fine line between gentle encouragement to undergo a test and coercion to do it, radiology staff tread this line day-in, day-out. We support nervous patients through tests but still give options to the hesitant. It is based on strict laws of consent.

Patients ask the advice of the staff when they face dilemmas about pushing on through with a scan or procedure. The older generation do this regularly. But sometimes they can't; they lack capacity to either ask or understand. And sometimes decisions have to be made rapidly. When a patient has been a major trauma or are bleeding rapidly from somewhere, there isn't time to have a conversation. You need to act in the patient's best interests.

This decision making process in determining the right test for an older patient is known as the 'Grandma Test'—would an average sensible person want this for their grandmother? You want compassionate care in addition to rigorous exploration of investigational and therapeutic options. You want neither over-investigation nor under-investigation. You want neither over-treatment nor under treatment.

I reject the calls of the 'everything must be done' brigade. These are often the younger relatives who call for every specialist to be consulted, every test under the sun to be performed and every treatment option tried. They reject pragmatism. They reject suggestions of futility. They do this through a misguided sense of propriety, possibly driven by guilt.

I'm not heartless: I'm anything but. It is just that 'Doing everything' fails the Grandma Test. Coercing a vulnerable and poorly individual into having fruitless tests is the opposite of caring. All medical investigations should be for the benefit of the individual patient. We certainly shouldn't be causing discomfort, inconvenience and suffering without any gain.

Sometimes it isn't the patient or their family but the medical team who are calling for a tranche of tests. This can be for a variety of reasons. Usually they haven't thought through what they are proposing for the patient. The answer to this is simply spelling out the reality of the situation. Sometimes the medical team are practising defensive medicine to avoid being sued: this is usually poor practice and can be safely omitted.

Just once in a while, the scan won't change any management decisions but is for prognostic purposes—as we'll see in Rule #59, this is the weakest of indications. One example of this radiological prognostication that I've seen a few times is scanning the terminally ill—an abominable practice that I'll take no part in (see Rule #64).

In all these circumstances, the radiologist should be bold. Scans that are not in the patient's best interests, scans that fail the Grandma Test should be rejected. As you'll see in the next Rule (#16), this is one place that a radiologist can legitimately say 'no' to a scan and always be correct.

Chapter 16
Rule #16 / / Be Damned Careful When Saying An Outright 'No'

The hardest part about being a radiologist is knowing when not to do something, when to say no. The clinician has seen the patient, you haven't. But if the most appropriate clinician hasn't seen the patient, feel free to say no. See Rules #13 & 15.

—

UK radiologists used to be gatekeepers. When I was in short medical trousers each hospital had one CT and one MRI scanner if they were lucky. Getting a scan was near impossible. Getting an *urgent* scan was laughable. We joked that the urgent scan requests had to be signed in the blood of the requesting doctor.

Before I became radiologist, a wiser and older radiologist told me 90% of the job at that time was 'sitting in the dark, telling people to 'eff off'. Sadly by the time I became a radiologist, telling other people to 'eff off was starting to become unacceptable. Clearly I missed the glory years.

Whilst only partially true, it was a necessity. On a good day we would scan twenty patients. CT scanners took longer to produce the images than it took to look at them. MRI was so slow that there was a risk that patients could develop metastatic disease during the scan.

One of my old bosses was known hospital-wide as 'Dr No'. It wasn't that she was an evil mastermind or had a rubber arm or anything. She would simply fix the quivering junior doctor with an unblinking stare, say a firm, "No" and that was that. No other words were necessary. It was a single word sentence. Moments later the request form was in shreds in the dustbin, providing the cue for the requesting doctor to exit apologetically.

This gate keeping role has virtually evaporated in the UK. The investigational chocolate box is wide open. Clinicians can help themselves to as many scans as they like, as often as they like, wherever they like. Radiologists rarely refuse. It actually takes longer to say no to a scan than do it. Which is all manner of wrong, of course.

© The Author(s), under exclusive license to Springer Nature Switzerland AG 2021
P. McCoubrie, *The Rules of Radiology*, https://doi.org/10.1007/978-3-030-65229-6_16

Some people say that better access to scans meets an unmet clinical need. Doing more scans is therefore better clinical practice. However I cannot shake the feeling that we are doing more and more scans and finding less and less. Pre-test probability means absolutely nothing in modern clinical practice. Our glorious diagnostic service is becoming a screening service.

We were told recently that scans looking for cancer should have positive pick up rate of around 3%. We laughed. And then we realised they were serious. Then our heads slowly slumped into our hands.

You see, radiologists don't mind normal scans. They are quick and easy. I must admit that after the umpteenth normal scan, my heart paradoxically sinks slightly. On one hand, I'm truly glad that there is nothing wrong with people. On the other hand, my job is to find abnormalities. When scan after scan is curiously free of disease, repetitive pronouncement of normality starts to feel hollow.

Furthermore if you were 99% certain that a particular scan or procedure is going to be normal before doing it then there is justified irritation. Also if you are 99% certain of the diagnosis before you start, it is waste-of-time-ogram. You haven't moved anything on. You haven't changed the medical management plan. You haven't helped the patient.

But being annoyed or wasting healthcare resources aren't the biggest problems. The problem relates to statistics. Specifically Bayesian statistics. The Rev Thomas Bayes discovered a few nuggets around 250 years ago that are still pertinent today.

When your disease prevalence drops to 3% then, even with a very accurate test like CT, most of your positive results are erroneous. Technically speaking your post-test probability is so low that most positive results are false positive. I won't labour the nerdy stats angle but if you understand about likelihood ratios and so forth, you'll know this is true.

These investigational red herrings are a positive menace. One of the big problems is the need for confirmatory tests. You have to somehow sort the true positive wheat from the false positive chaff. Further tests entail more expense, risk and incovenience for all concerned.

If most positive results result in yet another diagnostic wild goose chase, it is inevitable that radiologists and clinicians start to lose faith in the test. Radiologist doubt their findings. Clinicians don't believe abnormal test results. Hence the test stops functioning as a test. It is still as accurate as ever but it is why screening tests aren't accurate.

The long and short of this statistical reality is that radiologists have a real imperative to reject scans that look like a waste of time. It might seem ironic but saying a firm and simple 'No' can be doing the patient and the clinician a big favour in the long run.

I advocate that we need to all become a little more 'Dr No'. We need to differentiate clinical demand from clinical need and support the latter. We need the sense to recognise bovine excrement and the conviction to denounce it. Sometimes we radiologists *do* know best.

Radiologists need to regain a little fire in their bellies. We should be bold and decisive, borderline unreasonable. As George Bernard Shaw said, "The reasonable man adapts himself to the world: the unreasonable one persists in trying to adapt the world to himself. Therefore all progress depends on the unreasonable man."

Being borderline unreasonable needs to be tempered. It is tempting to shriek, "My machines!!! My machines!!!" and deny scans on a whim. It isn't helpful to nihilistically claim "It's a waste of time" to every request. It isn't warranted to grill every requesting clinician about irrelevant fine detail, demanding to know the serum rhubarb and urinary custard concentrations to 3 decimal places.

I have had many people ask how can I know if the scan needs doing if I haven't seen the patient myself. Surely I should just take the clinician's word for it? Well two big problems there. Huge stumbling blocks. They are assumptions that don't work anymore.

The first problem is that I have no assurances that the requesting clinician has seen and fully assessed the patient. I've had detailed conversations about the need for scanning a patient who, it later transpires, hasn't even arrived in the hospital. Often someone has seen and assessed the patient, just it is rarely the person I am talking to. I certainly won't tolerate requests from a surgeon to scan the patient before they have seen the patient themselves.

The second problem is more a philosophical one. This is the notion that is easier to do tests rather than not. A strategically-shaved simian with a stethoscope can click on computerised options, asking for a boatload of tests, spending £1000 s in less than a minute. Doing tests, prescribing treatment and performing therapeutic procedures is an active process. You are being seen to do something.

Doing nothing and doing it deliberately is possible. But doing it well is one of the hardest things in medical practice. It needs the wisdom that comes from years of expertise, a library-worth of knowledge and effective communication skills. In years gone by, there would be beard stroking and clicking of tongues, followed by a period of hawk-like observation and masterly inactivity.

Nowadays the beards may be less fulsome than our forefathers but there are several terms that mean subtle variations of the same thing. 'Conservative management' is a phrase that, essentially, means easing off the investigational accelerator pedal and keeping treatment low-key. 'Active surveillance' indicates no treatment but keeping an investigational eye on proceedings. The most minimal is 'watchful waiting' which means do nothing and only treat symptoms if and when they arise.

The natural temptation to over-investigate and over-treat is now officially recognised. There are all manner of official initiatives to investigate lightly. Guidelines about appropriateness of tests are widespread. These are notionally written to guide clinicians but it is an open secret that they are explicitly written with a view to reducing unnecessary tests.

Similar plans are now widespread amongst hospital inpatients. It is common to hear about 'ceilings of care' and 'treatment escalation plans', particularly in the frail or those with limited treatment options. This is enlightened behaviour. It makes explicit the goals of investigation and treatment. With such forethought, unwarranted testing is prevented at source.

I hope I've explained the very real legitimacy of refusing scans. I won't lie; we radiologists often get it wrong. That is because the gatekeeping role is hard. It takes years of experience to effectively discriminate between scans that really need doing and those that really don't need doing.

I actually decline very few scans in reality. My axioms about accepting scans are fairly simple. I do insist that the patient should have been seen and fully assessed by the most appropriate person. Sometimes this is asking for a senior opinion, sometimes this is asking for a different speciality. I think this is reasonable. Thereafter I accept the request if it bears evidence of logical thought. That is it. Nothing complex. But you would be surprised by how many requests bear no evidence of logical thought.

Chapter 17
Rule #17 / / Don't Study Surrogates

Many radiologists spend hours studying, with great precision, that which does not matter. Cut to the chase; study important primary outcomes, irrespective of how hard it. Anything else is lazy.

———

This might be a slightly surprising Rule. It is the only Rule about research amidst a sea of Rules about clinical practice. It is here for a good reason: this Rule is about stamping out lame research.

You might think that this is a forlorn venture and you'd probably be right. Merely railing against an unstoppable tsunami of woeful studies is unlikely to change anything.

Poor research is a blight on my beautiful speciality. I feel almost a moral duty to point at this dirty stain on radiology's good name. I will admit that I am working myself up into a minor lather about this. I will explain.

Radiology has been around for a while but if you're not familiar with the radiological academic canon, you might be surprised. You might imagine that there is a wealth of evidence behind the basics of what we do. But no, radiology is not a castle built on rock. Our scholastic foundations are pretty much loose sand. The sum total of 120+ years of academic literature is fairly flimsy, if truth be told.

This isn't a random assertion. I've been involved in a major national guidelines which entailed detailed literature searches. I know that, ironically, the basics of our speciality have very little evidence behind them. This is in spite of an on-going massive expansion in the published literature.

For example, it was over 20 years after mammography screening began in the UK before anyone showed that it saved lives. Even then, some authors insist that it actually doesn't: it remains controversial. Even more basic, consider the use of the humble chest x-ray looking for pneumonia. There is very little evidence behind it's use despite it being performed innumerable times over the last century.

© The Author(s), under exclusive license to Springer Nature Switzerland AG 2021
P. McCoubrie, *The Rules of Radiology*, https://doi.org/10.1007/978-3-030-65229-6_17

Radiology is one of the most fast-moving medical specialities. The speciality is barely recognisable from 40 years ago. The scanners from even 20 years ago are so antiquated as to seem like alien artefacts. Those using scanners over 10 years old are not castigated, just pitied.

A normal state of affairs in radiology is the fairly brisk adoption of something new with variable amounts of evidence following several years later. This isn't because we are reckless cavaliers. The new stuff (techniques, scanners, kit) that we are using is of proven safety just not of proven benefit. On the coal-face, we can see immediate benefits and thus start using it. Or at least we strongly suspect there is a benefit and are prepared to give it a whirl.

Sometimes we take the new thing up only to drop it like a hot potato; it just doesn't work in practice. Sometimes we use it in parallel to standard practice; it slowly finds a clinical niche. Sometimes it rapidly supplants existing practice; the new vanquishes the old. Occasionally research studies are then performed to prove the gut-feeling of a benefit. Often no study is done. Sometimes observational data is gathered. Advances in radiology are frequently evidence-light.

Radiology is highly tech-driven. It is constantly evolving. Actually, mutating might be a better way to describe it. Evolution is slow-paced and often minor, each improvement making the species better able to survive. Mutation is rapid, sudden, strange and often short-lived. There is no guarantee that any given mutation will be of benefit.

The first radiology research sin relates to this. This type of study describes a technological development but without any real attempt to look at benefits for patients. The radiology journals are peppered with these. Terribly impressive glossy pictures. Majestic graphs and tables. Until you read the paper is based on scanning four patients.

This type of publication gets up my nose as it is unabashed one-upmanship. We've got a new fancy scanner and you haven't. The authors are, in essence, thumbing their nose at you and saying, 'nyah-nyah'. This sort of paper should be printed on soft, strong and thoroughly absorbent paper. That way you have a chance of getting at least transient satisfaction from it.

Another type of radiological malfeasance is the retrospective review. These are rife in the radiological literature, largely as they methodologically easy. Don't get me wrong, they have a role. But it is a minor role as they are inherently flawed. Any retrospective study is riddled with uncontrolled bias.

Some bias is obvious, some bias is subtle but you can't remove it. It is intrinsic to retrospective data. Now I've only a shred of academic kudos. At most, I've left a few footprints on the hallowed turf of academe. But I've done more than my fair share of academic reviews; a few hundred papers have passed under my critical gaze. As a direct result I abhor retrospective reviews.

The irritating issue with retrospective studies is that authors are seemingly blind to bias. I could be kind and grant them ignorance. But I suspect it is largely wilful. Therefore the whole premise of the study is undermined and any conclusions asserted from the data are weakened. If I had a penny for paper I've read that contained an assertion based on biased data, I'd have about £5.67.

I have sympathy. Doing prospective studies is almost impossible these days. Certainly in the UK, the paperwork and processes are particularly hidebound. The laudable intent was to ensure that only methodologically-sound prospective studies are performed. But the unintended side-effect has been to strangle small-scale studies.

The motivation to perform academic studies is to, ultimately, improve the care we provide to our patients. Or so you would have thought. The complete cynic in me would argue that motivation is mainly about self-advancement. The motif of 'publish or die' is alive and kicking in academic radiology circles. All of our radiology registrars are pretty much mandated to indulge in research.

However, academic fame is near impossible now. The low hanging fruit of research have been picked. The days are long gone where a seminal paper could be achieved in a single afternoon with only a bottle of contrast, a long needle and a nervous-looking student volunteer. The profusion of radiology journals now means that any academic achievement is instantly diluted to homeopathic levels.

It is difficult to stay up to date with the literature. Some radiologists are very on the ball, making time in their busy schedules, avidly reading the latest journals cover-to-cover. At the other end of the spectrum is the radiologist who passively accumulates teetering stacks of journals, with strata spanning several years, mostly still pristine in their wrappers.

Most of us are in the middle; we read articles of interest but skim the rest. I'll admit mild work-related monomania but even I have a modest pile of unread journals skulking under my desk. Every time I stretch and stub my toe on it, I feel a pang of pedagogical remorse.

Back to the Rule—an exhortation to improve research in radiology. If you plan research then you must measure important outcomes. For example, if you are looking at a life-saving treatment, you must measure lives saved by that treatment. No argument. It may be difficult but if you've got eyes in your head and fingers on your hands then it can be measured.

There are always reasons for measuring surrogate outcomes. You measure improvement on the scan as a surrogate for improved survival, as an example. The main excuse is expediency or practicability: 'it wouldn't be feasible to measure anything else' and, 'measuring secondary outcomes is common practice', the investigators plea. Truth is that it is often laziness. Measuring surrogates is easier.

Your study should also be set up to gather enough data to be able to draw firm conclusions. Obviously a pilot study is a different matter, deliberately small scale to guide a subsequent larger project. But I'm astonished by how many pilot studies are submitted to journals. I'm totally flabbergasted by how many of the damnable things are actually published.

I therefore reject small-scale studies with surrogate outcomes. They cheapen and demean the condition you are studying. It is an insult to the patient. By doing a poor quality study you don't advance knowledge. You induce uncertainty, you muddy the evidence and therefore impede knowledge. When I read 'further study is recommended' I can't help thinking 'why the hell didn't you do it then?'.

The worst case scenario is that your study is flawed and your findings are just plain wrong. An erroneous statement of causation is hard to refute as, scientifically speaking, proving a negative hypothesis is almost impossible. Especially when it is a link with something common and something rare.

Here is an *reductio ad absurdam* example. There is a theoretical risk of endocarditis in high-risk patients after barium enema. An official statement dictated that these patients should be given preventative antibiotics. So a sarcastic radiologist wrote a letter to a learned journal where they opined that patients undergoing a barium enema should wear a tea-cosy on their head. They reasoned that if a helicopter fell from the sky onto the patient, it would provide cranial protection.

They reasoned you can't be too safe and considered it immaterial that (i) this had never happened and (ii) the tea-cosy provided uncertain protection. Funnily enough, the official advice was withdrawn shortly afterwards. This shows good quality evidence is everything. We are lost without it.

Chapter 18
Rule #18 / / Avoid 'Interesting' Cases

They aren't. They've asked everyone else already. And, no, they don't have a clue either.

—

Picture the scene. You are sat merrily beavering away at your day job when a colleague sidles up and, with a slight waggle of the eyebrows, asks if they can they can show you something interesting. Normally your ears prick up. Chances are that it is probably amusing and a little outré. Unless the individual is unsavoury or you have a pressing deadline, you welcome this distraction.

However, when a radiologist sidles up to another radiologist and asks the same question then it is very very different. The comedic facial expression may be the same but they aren't usually wanting to show you something amusing. Contrary to popular belief, few radiologists keep unusual or amusing x-rays. I have literally zero x-rays of foreign bodies that have been inserted into body cavities. Of course I don't. It is all CT these days.

Occasionally the colleague is sharing a 'good' case, one where the appearances are particularly striking or 'classic'. The medical jargon for this is 'pathognomomic' which is nothing to do with paths or gnomes but of Greek origin, meaning 'characteristic of a specific disease'. A classic case may well be textbook-worthy, or even better than those in the textbooks. These are definitely keepers; 'prize rabbits' as my grandfather used to say.

There is a curious pride or low-grade excitement in looking at such scans. Radiologists want to share this excitement with their colleagues. If they work in a good radiology department then this kind of interaction is common. The best departments have this formalised with regular case review meetings. As a rule of thumb, the better the department, the more regular the meetings. Radiologists that work in a department with daily or weekly meetings should count their blessings; they are lucky little sausages.

© The Author(s), under exclusive license to Springer Nature Switzerland AG 2021   69
P. McCoubrie, *The Rules of Radiology*, https://doi.org/10.1007/978-3-030-65229-6_18

We radiologists love the thrill of the investigational chase. We are greedy for it; positively lustful. Ask us to hunt for the diagnosis in a poorly patient and we will go at it like a dog at a still-warm cooked chicken. We prize the rare clinch, the diagnosis we pull out of the bag despite scant evidence. We hunt mercilessly for anatomical snippets, the faintest hints of disease and then try to pull it together into a coherent diagnosis. In fact, the more others have tried and failed, the more we revel in the challenge.

Confidently making a rare or unusual diagnosis is the Holy Grail of radiology. It isn't that we do this for plaudits, although it is a strange radiologist that is truly averse to well-earned praise. The internal glow of diagnostic success is all we seek. It is a reward in itself. It lasts far longer than fine words from colleagues. But there is a downside to this overt focus on the diagnostic process. We forget about the patient, their wants, needs and desires. This can lead to Pyrrhic diagnostic triumphs.

One of my proudest diagnostic moments was diagnosing an incredibly rare condition on a bone scintigram (Erdheim-Chester disease). The crowning glory was that this diagnosis came after the patient had undergone twenty-five fruitless years of intense investigation by others. I was, dear reader, immensely proud. Borderline insufferable. But three months after my triumph, the patient sadly died from their disease. All of a sudden I didn't feel so clever anymore.

I often describe radiologists as being the Sherlock Holmes of the medical world. Of course, Sir Arthur Conan Doyle based Holmes on one of the foremost diagnosticians of the time, Dr Joseph Bell, an Edinburgh surgeon. Conan Doyle worked as a junior doctor under Bell in 1877, well before radiology existed. It was Bell's legendary close clinical observation and logical extrapolation of these observations that so inspired the character of Holmes. And indeed the latter-day TV character from *House M.D.*, famed for his diagnostic abilities, is acknowledged to be based on Holmes' character.

The parallel between Holmes (or House) and radiology works on other levels. Like Holmes, we love a difficult case. Give us the choice of straightforward or fiendishly difficult and we'll always want to have a crack at the latter. Also akin to the famed detective, we can be deeply antisocial during the investigative process; utterly intolerant of interruptions, coming down hard on even the faintest wisp of distraction. Our equivalent of Dr Watson writing up the case is us keeping a note of the case for later review, reference and demonstration to others. But we draw the line at smoking a pipe, playing a violin and intravenous injection of cocaine in the radiology department.

Radiology is almost entirely visual. So we literally do show each other cases in a way that clinicians cannot. Clinicians used to show off their patients, wheeling them into packed medical lecture theatres to show off their physical signs and to ask them to tell their stories. Most patients felt distinctly uncomfortable with being a prize exhibit but some did volunteer. Some patients are still keen to be involved in education but clinicians rarely now feel comfortable metaphorically twisting the arms of patients. Such once mighty Medical Grand Rounds are now just Death by Powerpoint instead.

Recording details about individual cases has a long history. Probably the earliest was Hippocrates who detailed some pretty spectacular examples around 400BC. The great-grandfather of modern clinical method, William Osler, famously instructed students, "Observe, record, tabulate, communicate". He did just that, becoming the premier medical educator of his time. Sigmund Freud, famed psychiatrist, took the case report to new heights, writing whole books about single patients.

Thus for hundreds of years the medical literature was largely full of learning points from cases reports and the odd case series. Osler famously cut his academic teeth with a number of case series, largely based on necropsies he had performed himself. At that time negative patient feedback was largely presented in the post mortem room. Diseased organs were removed at necropsy and then pickled in a jar. Such preserved specimens were then the primary way to learn about disease.

The 'path pot' enjoyed over 150 years of educational primacy. It ruled over textbooks of the time. It was a common feature in medical exams. Many generations of medical students have frozen with fear when a sealed glass jar containing an unidentifiable specimen was passed across the examination table.

A good specimen was a highly prized object. A rare specimen was even more exalted. Even as late as the 1980s, a medical institute was of no standing without an extensive medical museum. The more prestigious the institute, the more bizarre and wide-ranging was the collection of medical oddities. For example, the Royal College of Surgeon's Hunterian Collection in London spans four centuries and contains over 3500 specimens. However, such specimen collection was free of ethical considerations. At the time of writing, the inclusion of 'The Irish Giant' (Charles Byrne's eight foot skeleton) in this collection remains distinctly controversial.

In the last thirty years, this obsessive and slightly morbid collection of chunks of diseased human tissue has been supplanted with radiological imaging. Of course a scan isn't as dramatic as, say, a pickled adult human hand. But it has the advantage of not being reliant on the patient being dead first. Plus you don't need a huge physical museum. The average computer's hard drive will hold several thousand cases. Connect that to the internet and you have an on-line museum that anyone can visit. The modern battle is now between slick commercial versions and Free Open Access Medical Education (FOAMed) sites.

These on-line radiological repositories are fulfilling the same duties as Osler did the late 19th C. They are full of 'classic cases' for education and edification. This is different to the 'interesting' case. The latter are one of two things. Either they are particularly bizarre or gross cases, the radiological equivalent of a bearded lady. There isn't much to learn but they are interesting to look at. Or they are cases where no one has a clue what is going on.

Radiologists have good reasons to be trepidatious about the latter cases. You get involved with the best of intentions, usually when a colleague asks for a second pair of eyes. After all, you want to help the patient. But, before you know it, you are embroiled. Your name is also on the radiology report as either an addendum or 'discussed with'.

Except rarely does anything good come out of such case reviews. These are cases where the published evidence is of no use. This stuff isn't in the textbooks. It is 'emergent practice' (i.e. flying by the seat of their pants). Ninety percent of the time the outcome is 'I've no idea either'. In around nine percent is a partial outcome along the lines of 'I don't know but could be x, y, or z'. Just occasionally you are the one percent. You chip in something valuable; your colleague slaps you firmly on the shoulder and progress is made. For the other ninety-nine percent of cases the only benefactor is your colleague who feels less bad.

However interesting cases can end badly. Before you know it you are trouble for merely helping out. You end up being cited on a complaint or lawsuit (I speak from bitter experience). Being a Good Samaritan in radiology has few tangible benefits and is a definite double-edged sword. Approach interesting cases with extreme caution.

Chapter 19
Rule #19 // Beware The 'Fit 90 Year Old'

There is no such thing.

———

A radiologist hearing the phrase 'fit 90 year old' will smile in recognition. It is a cliché you've heard a thousand times before. It is also a weasel phrase as, frankly, it is borderline dishonest. The use of such a phrase is a marker of a fairly ballsy clinician; one who is prepared to bend the truth to achieve their goals. They need a scan, so anything goes, eh? No. Honesty is a strict moral line over which doctors shouldn't cross. Somehow radiology requests seem to be exempt. Normally scrupulous doctors have no qualms about producing minor works of fiction in the clinical details section (see Rule #36).

You might be mildly shocked by my assertion that such an innocuous statement is somehow immoral. However such a phrase is palpable nonsense. The majority of ninety year olds are physically frail. Dementia is an ever-present undercurrent in old age, 30% have a formal diagnosis and many more are playing without a full deck. They are literally nearing the end of life; life expectancy at ninety is around four years. To put this in context, being ninety has worse survival prospects than seven of the top ten cancers.

It is actually pretty rare to find anyone over ninety that is truly fit. And when I say truly fit, I mean that they can run, skip and dance like a normal adult. Ok, maybe not dance. I can't dance like a normal adult; never could. Yet we radiologists are told about these mythical creatures on a regular basis. You would imagine, from what we are told, that the hospital is crammed with lithe senior citizens in lycra, near-centennials jogging around the wards, great-grandfathers doing press-ups in the foyer. Fitness in nonagenarians is a relative concept. 'Fit for 90' is entirely different and much more appropriate.

As a doctor you want what you think is best for your patients. Normally this entails asking others to play a role. Which normally happens like clockwork. But occasionally others don't want to join in on the fun. Sometimes this is sloth,

© The Author(s), under exclusive license to Springer Nature Switzerland AG 2021
P. McCoubrie, *The Rules of Radiology*, https://doi.org/10.1007/978-3-030-65229-6_19

sometimes this is rationing of a resource, sometimes they frankly disagree with your course of actions. So you bargain with them. This is nothing new. Doctors have been horse-trading on behalf of their patients since Imhotep was a lad. Over the centuries we've moved from referrals arriving on a papyrus scroll to electronic referrals. But if you want to get something done quickly, the face-to-face conversation or telephone call is still best.

There is a specific aspect of this bargaining process that is predominantly found amongst hospital inpatients. This is the processes of 'buffing' and 'turfing'. These concepts were popularised over forty years ago in Samuel Shem's 1978 novel '*House of God*' and are still going strong to this day.

'Buffing' is making a patient look better on paper than they are in reality. Sometimes this is to persuade other doctors (radiologists included) to do something that they would think twice about if they met the patient face to face. Other times it is purely about making it look like the patient is improving due to your diligent care whereas, in reality, no such improvement has occurred. And every so often it is the opposite.

'Turfing' is persuading another team to take over care of the patient. Mostly this is a genuine plea; a patient with a rigid abdomen should be under the general surgical team, even if they were initially admitted with a nosebleed. As a prelude to an attempt at a turf, the patient must be fully buffed. Then the successful turfer tries to 'sell' their patient to their target team, engaging every and all tactics as necessary.

Some specialities are famously hard-nosed. Neurosurgeons are famously picky about patients that they will accept into their precious beds. The patient can be neither too old nor too young. If the patient is not sick enough then they won't take them. But if they are too sick, then they won't taken them either. If they've only had a CT, they need an MRI. If they've had an MRI, they need an MRI with contrast. Turfing to neurosurgery is a famously tough sell.

Asking a radiologist to do a scan on a patient involves the same processes. Any possible difficulties are air-brushed over. The saintly, white-haired great-grandmother that is sold to you as needing a scan turns out to be Granny-zilla: rearing up out of her bed, aggressively delirious, prone to roaring, and eager to bite staff with her single remaining upper left incisor. I see a great number of requests that start "Previously fit and well ..." but omit minor details such as Grade IV heart failure, lower limb amputation or dense hemiplegia. Often there is a capricious mix of all three with a light dusting of dementia on top.

Hence when a junior doctor opens their spiel with 'this fit 90 year old', we know what is really coming next. You are being sent someone who is going to struggle. Just wheeling them into the department makes them distressed. They certainly don't like CT scanners and don't even think about putting them anywhere near an MRI machine. Oh and don't sedate them either. Paradoxical agitation is a very real phenomenon and no fun for anyone.

I should point out that radiologists aren't ageist. Quite the reverse. We generally love older people. They are normally unfailingly polite, immensely stoic, endlessly thankful and reliably punctual. In other words the elderly are usually model patients. So what is the problem, I hear you cry. The problem is complex.

The first part of this is that old people do not like having scans. The older and frailer they are, the less they like them. The more detailed and lengthy the scan, the less they like them. The more invasive, the more preparation that is required, the less they like them. The frail elderly are also vulnerable. They cannot easily consent to (or refuse) investigations. So we radiologists have to make a judgement call—we apply the 'Grandma Test' (see Rule #15).

It is for this reason we radiologists are naturally reluctant to scan the frail elderly. We know what the scan entails and watch them having to endure it. We just aren't into elder abuse. Now I don't think you'd get many clinicians holding up their hand there. It is just that clinicians don't see what their patients have to go through. They don't see Mr Smith having an attack of the screaming habdabs, needing twenty minutes of gentle coaxing to finish the scan you'd just started.

The second part of this is a rapid increase in investigation of those in extreme old age. Scanning someone over 100 years old used to be a distinct novelty but it now barely raises an eyebrow. There are undeniably more old people than ever before. The number of people over eighty-five is projected to double between 2015 and 2035 in most developed countries. But scanning is increasing disproportionately. In just seven years our department saw an 50% increase in activity in those aged over ninety. CT is hit most—we are doing 120% more. Whilst some might argue that more radiological investigation equates to better medical care, this is not necessarily so. This isn't simple demographic changes, clinical practice has changed.

Perhaps part of this rise in investigation of old folk is a correction of outdated and paternalistic ageism. Attitudes were different a medical generation ago. Disease in old age was treated symptomatically and was minimally investigated, if at all. It wasn't long ago that hypertension in those over 80 wasn't considered worth treating and pneumonia was 'an old man's friend'. Although, to be honest, both examples are not quite as black and white as they seem.

The third issue is that the goals of care in this patient cohort are different. Towards the end of life, medical care is predominantly palliative—improving quality of life, maintaining function and maximising comfort. Consequently a different radiological approach is required. This involves treading a narrow path. On one hand, you don't want to under-investigate symptoms and risk missing treatable disease. On the other hand, you don't want to over-investigate and cause needless distress and suffering. This balancing act is complex. It needs careful thought and discussion.

And while Geriatricians are experts are doing this, the average surgeon or physician doesn't necessarily think this way. Certainly the junior doctors on the ward don't always acknowledge the frail elderly as any different to their other patients. We need to think about 'light touch' investigation: doing the minimum number of investigations that are as minimally invasive as possible but aimed at providing maximum symptomatic benefit.

This could be termed 'palliative radiology', quite different to our normal cura-tive investigational paradigm. Such an approach has much to be commended; paradoxically improving patient care by doing fewer tests. It is a nudge of the investigational pendulum, putting it back into proper alignment.

Chapter 20
Rule #20 / / Counteract Misjudgement

Staff and patients make snap judgements about you. Overcompensate. Dress smarter and behave more professionally than you think you should.

—

Radiologists are usually pretty robust types. You'll find few delicate flowers in the radiology garden. Climbing up the medical career ladder needs a thick hide to withstand the metaphorical attacks that inevitably occur during postgraduate training (Fig. 20.1). On the flip side, I don't know many radiologists who are emotionally dead, impervious to the opinions of others, bereft of normal social graces. Underneath a radiologist's mental armour usually beats the heart of normal human.

We aren't needy but, being normal human beings, we don't particularly like being disliked. More specifically, we don't being disliked for no particular reason. I should specify that radiologists don't need praise. You don't go into radiology if you want to be loved. Praise rarely comes our way; you learn that on day one of radiology school. So even if you want it, you are not going to get it. So you have to make do without it.

Radiologists meet a lot of patients but for a brief period of time. There is not enough time to form a anything resembling a therapeutic relationship. There are some patients that I've scanned a number of times and the handshakes are a little firmer, the jokes a bit chummier, and the conversation a bit more direct. But they form probably less than 1 in 100 of the people I scan.

It is similar with staff. The hospital I work in employs 8000 staff. Our department has over 350 staff. Aside from my colleagues, I form a good relationship with only a handful of clinicians. There are over 400 consultants and many more junior doctors. There seem to be an awful lot of anaesthetists these days; they are the modern day medical mafia, seemingly holding the whole hospital to ransom. Nothing, it seems, can happen without the assent of a coterie of 'those who pass gas'. My vision of a modern anaesthetic department has a Marlon Brando-esque

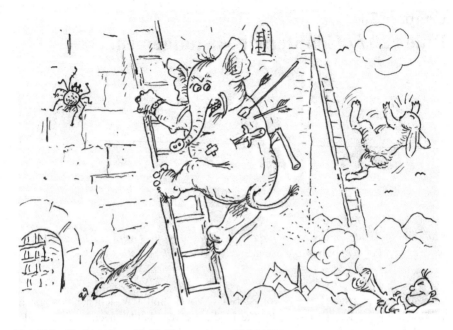

Fig. 20.1 Climbing the medial ladder requires a thick hide

boss anaesthetist at its shadowy heart, clad in gold-embroidered black scrubs, surrounded by burly operating department assistants.

Anyway, due to this permanent brevity of interaction, we get used to people making snap judgements about us. Others cast their eyes over you and within milliseconds have formed opinions just on your appearance. All your initial actions, verbal and non-verbal, are judged. We know that first impressions tend to last well after you get to know someone. This is a feature of all cultures, all races, all parts of the globe, whether we like it or not. To make snap judgements is to be human. Actually, to be strictly honest, making snap judgements is more chimp than human.

It is fashionable to talk about the 'inner chimp'. Many psychologists have cashed in on our improved understanding of the ways that we think as individuals, as groups, and as societies. The parts of the brain involved in forming initial impressions are similar in structure and function to our close cousin, *Pan troglodytes*, the chimpanzee. These structures, the limbic system, are a key part of rapid responses that ensure survival: the fight-or-flight reflex actions. They are also ancient in their ontology, being widespread amongst mammals, birds and reptiles. Heck, there is evidence that even dinosaurs had limbic systems.

These largely subconscious if primitive feelings are often called system 1 or type 1 thinking. They have a complex relationship with the more rational and nuanced output of our human brain (system 2 or type 2 thinking). Our existence is, in essence, a tussle between these two thought processes. We have careful and deliberate thought from our neocortex which is often at odds with the base reflex thoughts of our old mammal brain.

A summary of type 1 and 2 thinking is beyond the scope of this chapter. It took Nobel Prize-winning Profession Daniel Kahneman 467 pages to briefly summarise the major points in his 2011 epic 'Thinking, Fast and Slow'. The cruxes of this tome are that (i) judgement is often flawed, (ii) most people are blind to this and (iii) people have too much confidence in human judgement.

Trusting one's gut instincts is deeply ingrained. Our brains are hard-wired to make rapid judgements via system 1. You can't avoid it even if you are aware of it. Whether we like it or not, our subconscious brain is constantly sizing people up. When you see an attractive person you've formed a favourable impression of them within less than 1/10th of the time it takes to blink. On a different occasion, despite the attempts to tell yourself otherwise, your amygdala rapidly hijacks your neocortex and forms a negative opinion of an ugly person in a few milliseconds. In other words, people know that they shouldn't judge a book by its cover but cannot help themselves.

Although first impressions are generally accurate, people are easily fooled. The notion that people can spot liars is largely false. You don't need to be an Oscar-winning actor to convincingly fake emotion or spin a falsehood. Indeed, the history of the human race is littered with stories of people who have duped many people over many years. The medical world is absolutely full of them, exploiting various aspects of the human psyche. Snake-oil salesmen have always been with us, medical fraudsters have been doing it for several centuries.

The history of medical legislation and certification is largely a history of preventing charlatans pretending to be doctors. Many other healthcare professions have a similar history. And woe betide you if your standards slip. The General Medical Council and other similar bodies will happily strike you off for a one-off indiscretion. This doesn't stop a massive industry of quackery at the fringes of conventional medicine. Take homeopathy as an example, still alive and kicking where a rational species would have smothered it at birth.

Guilty admission here. Medics are trained to fake it. As part of communication skills training, for example, we are explicitly shown what an empathic doctor looks like, acts and says. The notion being that even if you aren't feeling empathic, you can trot out a close facsimile. It is done with a higher purpose—to help the patient. Does it matter if your doctor is truly empathic or is just very good at faking it? Probably not, so long as the patient gets what they need.

This is part of being a professional. In the few tender hours before work, your dog might have piddled in your shoes and the children might have deliberately smashed your favourite *Bagpuss* DVD but you have to turn up to work and pretend everything is fine. People talk about a professional mask and sometimes it does feel like that. Exuding bonhomie when you feel like thunder needs a strong degree of self-control. Radiating empathy when you actually don't feel like it needs a certain degree of professionalism.

I'm astonished by the minority of healthcare professionals who don't bother to hide their emotions. I think is absolutely essential. The purpose of a professional front is to hold your true feelings in check. Your moral duty is to treat everyone equally, irrespective of your mood. It is also your duty to offer equally good care irrespective of your affinity with the patient, be they beautiful or ugly, fat or slim, dim or bright, friendly or hostile, young or old, smelly or fragrant, disabled or able-bodied.

I know several radiologists who don't even pretend anymore. You know the type. The ones that are unsmiling and grouchy, the ones that everyone avoids, the ones that don't give a monkey's about anyone or anything. Is it that they are bad people who have no place as a healthcare professional? Are they merely products of a dysfunctional training? Could it be that they are perfectly competent but lack emotional intelligence? Or is it because they've been ground down by an exploitative healthcare system, leaving only a cynical husk behind? As ever, it is complex and probably a combination of these things.

So how do we combat this? Well, helpfully, the Rules of Radiology are here to provide guidance. First, you must dress appropriately smartly (see Rule #87). Next, you must always introduce yourself (see Rule #78). And, finally, always smile (see Rule #2). The rest is entirely up to you. It depends on the professional persona that you want to project and to what extent you want to project it. It also depends on knowing your own foibles, knowing the things that you do that can cause people to misjudge you.

Personally I've always aimed for a highly professional first ten seconds and then play the rest by ear. My personal style is to sit or stand up straight and look them in the eye when you greet them, making a clear display of giving them your full attention. I tend to proffer a firm handshake and a weak joke as an ice-breaker. I can't recommend the latter strategy to everyone. I know some mirthless types who wouldn't know a thrombosed haemorrhoid from olecranon bursitis. But if you can, please do. Jollity is highly therapeutic and has few side effects.

Chapter 21
Rule #21 / / There Is No Such Thing As A Radiological Emergency

If the patient has a cardiac arrest in the department it isn't strictly a radiological matter. Whilst it is polite to show an interest, they'd be honestly better off with the crash team. Otherwise, you should always finish your cuppa before the next task. Rushing things causes errors. Stay calm, stay safe (Fig. 21.1).

—

There are many reasons that medical graduates choose to sub-specialise in radiology, if you discount the obvious reasons of the glamour, an abiding love of radiation and an unquenchable thirst for knowledge of the innards of strangers. One strong influence has been the attraction of regular hours.

Certainly this was true twenty-odd years ago. When I was a registrar, radiology departments stirred reluctantly into life at 9am. The shutters came down at 5 pm on the dot whereupon the radiologists would promptly emerge from their darkened rooms, blinking into the afternoon light.

We were rarely called back. Out-of-hours services were scant. And out-of-hours was strictly 5.01 pm–08.59 am. The attitude was that virtually everything could wait until the next morning. Whilst this is still true in the vast majority of cases, then it was true because an out of hours scan in the pre-digital era was such a palaver.

There was none of this workstation-at-home business; it involved several phone calls and a schlep to the hospital. We didn't have specially trained staff—one or two radiographers covered the entire department. Doing a CT was a painful ordeal. The on-call radiographic staff often had to pull out the instruction book. 'Step one—press the big red button to switch the scanner on. Step two…'. Generally a single scan would take a minimum of a few hours.

This clunky system existed because it was an inherited pattern from traditional radiology practice. Radiology played little role in the treatment of an acutely ill patient. Apart from an x-ray or two, we had little to offer. I remember distinctly an elderly CT scanner from the late 1980s taking a full minute per slice. A head CT

© The Author(s), under exclusive license to Springer Nature Switzerland AG 2021
P. McCoubrie, *The Rules of Radiology*, https://doi.org/10.1007/978-3-030-65229-6_21

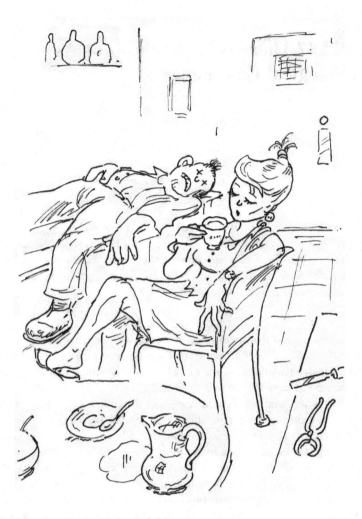

Fig. 21.1 Otherwise you should always finish your cuppa

took a minimum of 20 min. You needed a certain zen-like calmness when scanning sick patients. It simply couldn't be rushed.

Proper emergency CT was just not feasible until faster scanners became available in the mid-late 1990s. Before that time, scanning a critically ill patient was hazardous. You can monitor a patient in the scanner but you can't attend to them because of the radiation hazard to staff. CT scanners became known as 'the donut of death' as many patients expired mid-scan.

Modern radiological working patterns are unrecognisable from twenty years ago. Out-of-hours doesn't really exist anymore, we cover the emergency workload in a shift pattern. The scanners are zippy; whole body CT top-to-toe in twenty seconds. The scanners, as assets, are fully sweated, working a minimum 12 hr day.

None of this putting scans off because it is a faff. Getting a emergency scan done is routine, the systems are now slick.

The rate limiting step is now the radiologist. Processes are now so slick that scans are produced faster than we can report them. Despite this, pressure to do a 'quick' scan should be resisted (Rule #45) and reports should be considered (Rule #52).

This wholesale shift in working patterns is in response to increased demand. And because scans are readily available 24/7, we have become victims of our own success. The number of scans performed 5 pm–9 am has mushroomed. In just ten years, we locally have gone from five-ten scans to fifty. At a weekend, we'll easily scan 200 patients. Many of these scans are literally life-saving. Our Major Trauma Service is totally centred on rapid access to CT. CT scanners should now be called 'the polo mint of life'.

With this massive throughput of patients, both in and out-of-hours, there are going to be a few medical emergencies in the radiology department. It is inevitable. By pure chance, if you have a large number of people in any one place, some of them will fall ill. I remember running to a cardiac arrest on the coronary care unit but rather than it being a patient, it was a relative in the visitors room that had keeled over. Lucky place to have a cardiac arrest, I thought. And indeed he walked out of hospital a few weeks later.

Most of these cardiac arrests don't have such a happy ending. The success rate of resuscitation attempts is parlous. But, if you think about it, it isn't surprising. When most people drop down dead, there is a solid and irreversible reason. No amount of chest compressions, fancy drugs and electricity to the heart will change this.

Occasionally, just occasionally, someone arrests from something sudden but treatable. And this is where medical miracles occur—people being brought back from the dead. It is the Holy Grail of medicine. Hence a lot of time and effort goes into providing a slick resuscitation service in hospitals.

When you are young, these are tremendously exciting events where you get to yell 'Charging 360, stand clear' and no one laughs at you. But after a few months of charging around the hospital at the beck and call of the 'arrest bleep', it becomes quite routine. After several years of doing this, the adrenaline is long gone and you start to realise the human tragedy of it all.

Cardiac arrests, like childbirth, are messy and thoroughly undignified affairs. But unlike childbirth, there is no happy ending in around 90% of cases. It is quite the opposite. Not the way that most people would chose to shuffle off their mortal coil.

In the UK we simply call these 'cardiac arrests' or 'crash calls'. 'Crashing' is where things go suddenly and horribly awry on the heart rate-blood pressure-breathing side of things, short of actually stopping completely. I don't know why 'crashing' is a thing but it generally indicates that arrest will follow shortly unless something is done.

In the US, patients are said to 'code'. This is short for 'code blue' meaning cardiac arrest, one of several standardised colour-based communication codes. The only code I have seen used in the UK is 'code brown' but I am not sure that a patient soiling the bed is actually a medical emergency.

As a younger radiologist I was assiduously bang up-to-date on cardiopulmonary resuscitation (CPR) and Advanced Life Support (ALS). But I slowly became a bit frustrated. A propos of nothing they'd change the acronyms just to confuse matters. For example, electromechanical disassociation (EMD) became pulseless electrical activity (PEA). I also became a little peeved that you'd fail any assessment if you didn't repeat the precise mantra you'd just been taught. The mantra was usually a standardised approach based on How We've Always Done It, which I can never easily sign up to. It felt like a minor self-serving industry and I opted out.

Proper cardiac arrests in radiology departments are actually fairly rare. Most people keeling over are simply fainting, requiring nothing more than a lie down and pat on the wrist. If it is a prolonged faint, apply the same rules but add a cup of hot sugary tea and a biscuit. It is widely acknowledged that NHS tea has remarkably restorative powers. You won't find any of this in official guidelines or textbooks. However, I've seen patients being on the verge of admission to intensive care only to have the timely intervention of a strong cuppa and a few Custard Creams. After this restorative miracle the patient walked unaided out of the department just thirty minutes later.

Whenever someone properly arrests in the department, I beetle along and normally find a full-blown resuscitation attempt in motion. A crowd of enthusiastic youngsters are swarming over the patient, doing the needful. I began to realise that I was a positive hindrance. Arriving short of puff and wheezing, I was told it is apparently poor form to snatch the oxygen off the patient.

For this reason, radiologists are usually better hands-off rather than hands-on. Sure, they can pour oil on the troubled waters by pronouncing the graveness of the scenario, issuing soothing words to those getting their hands dirty, and singing 'Stayin' Alive' to ensure the correct beats-per-minute of the cardiac massage.

I'm not saying radiologists should ignore crash calls. Nope, we should wade in and confirm a lack of pulse, call for help and, if appropriate, start chest compressions. The trick is not to arrive first at a cardiac arrest. The first person is obliged to start the resuscitation attempt on their own. Solo resuscitation is a thorny business; much easier with several pairs of hands. If you start a solo attempt, you've no idea who else is en route and how long they'll be. If you do arrive first, whatever you do, don't be tempted to sneak back out again. You are bound to get seen doing so. And that is a difficult one to live down.

The major issue is becoming deskilled. To remain slick, you need to regularly plunge head-long into emergency situations, reviving the moribund, parrying the scythe of the Grim Reaper, and medically slamming shut the Pearly Gates. Our skills as radiologists lie elsewhere. Leave the medical heroics to someone else and step away. Patients are better off without gung-ho radiologists pretending they've still got it.

Chapter 22
Rule #22 / / If You Feel Resistance, Stop Pushing

This is the cardinal rule of interventional radiology. Same rule applies when cleaning one's external auditory meatus.

—

There is an old medical adage that say, 'There is no body cavity that cannot be reached with a 14 gauge needle and good strong arm' (from *The House of God*). This used to be entirely true. However the standard hypodermic needle is a mere 4 cm long so this doesn't work in today's much larger patients, even with a very strong arm. The bigger problem is 14G needle is about as thick as a knitting needle. Should you prang other structures en route to the chosen body cavity, harm will be done, questions will be asked. To be honest, there is little need for such chunky needles these days. 95% of procedures use much finer needles.

The origin of Rule #22 is simple. If you are a radiologist that performs interventional procedures, then you tend to see the human body as a series of tubes and hollow spaces into which a needle can be introduced. An interventional procedure that is going smoothly should meet with minimal resistance. The needle, wire and catheter should slide in as if buttered. Apart from, perhaps, bone biopsies; always a bit on the crunchy side, by all accounts.

The more delicate the procedure, the less resistance you should tolerate. It also depends a little on your background. They say a neuroradiologist manipulates their wire with their finger tips, an interventional radiologist manipulates their wire with their fingers and wrists, the vascular surgeon manipulates their wire with their shoulder.

The notion of resistance can be physical and mental. Obviously if your needle, wire or catheter fails to advance easily then for God's sake stop. Ramming it home is a good way to do some serious harm. But this Rule also applies to feeling behavioural resistance from others. It covers a whole load of situations that commonly arise in the radiology workplace. Before that perhaps I should explain a little more about interventional radiology (IR).

© The Author(s), under exclusive license to Springer Nature Switzerland AG 2021
P. McCoubrie, *The Rules of Radiology*, https://doi.org/10.1007/978-3-030-65229-6_22

The boundary between interventional and diagnostic radiology is a slightly burry one. Over thirty years ago, it was all just 'radiology'. It was just some radiologists were more needle-happy than others. Essentially, it is IR if it involves sticking anything more than an intravenous cannula into the patient. Although radiology began as a diagnostic speciality, soon radiologists began to dreaming of ways to fix matters that they'd just diagnosed.

Charles Dotter (the founding father of IR) performed his first deliberate angioplasty in 1964—the first was a benign accident during a diagnostic procedure in 1963. To put this in context, this was seven years before the first CT scanner took an hour to produce shonky brain images and a full thirteen years before the first MRI scanner took 5 h to produce a blurry outline of a thorax. And yet despite this heritage, IR still hasn't penetrated into the public consciousness. To be quite honest, the general public have little idea of what a radiologist does and even less idea of what an interventional radiologist is.

Accordingly, IR has tried to reinvent itself with catchy slogans and buzz words. 'Minimally-invasive surgery' is one that I'm not sure works—surgery is what surgeons do. IR has been painted as 'pinhole surgery', just like laparoscopic procedures have been popularised as 'keyhole surgery'. My immediate thought was they are pretty big pins, creating holes generally sufficient to thread a small hosepipe into.

Radiology is a little like Zaphod Beeblebrox, one of the antiheroes in Douglas Adam's *Hitchhiker's Guide to the Galaxy* series. Not that we are recklessly fond of cocktails that are the alcoholic equivalent of being mugged, no. In the UK, we have a single body but fully formed diagnostic and interventional heads. There is the future possibility of the two splitting off into separate bodies but, for the meanwhile, the common body is made up of a solid core of diagnostic radiology.

Different radiologists do different proportions of interventional and diagnostic work. There are radiologists, like myself, who are 100% diagnostic and don't do any of that stabby-stabby stuff. There are radiologists who are the complete opposite; everyday is needles from dawn to dusk and diagnostic radiology is merely a way to plan their radiological voodoo. Then, in the middle, there are plenty of two-headed radiologists who do a bit of both.

Of course, the hard-core interventionists take the mickey out of the soft-handed, effete diagnostic radiologists. So we dyed-in-the-wool diagnosticians tease the 'grumpy torque monkeys' that perform 'manual labour'. We diagnostic radiologists mock their work as 'plumbing' and their theatre scrubs as 'pyjamas'; they deride our foppish refusal to get our hands dirty.

Amongst this friendly banter there have been some classic jibes too. Similar to the allegorical gynaecologist who decorated their front hall through the letter box, there is the joke about the interventional radiologist who re-plumbed their house via the kitchen tap, all whilst the boiler was switched on. Not forgetting made-up IR procedures like the transanal laryngeal ablation or perurethral orchidopexy.

IR differs hugely across the world. In some countries, interventional procedures are performed by different specialities. For example, cardiologists have made cardiac intervention their own and some have expanded their vascular portfolio, probably because day-in, day-out intervention on the same two arteries of the heart gets a little tedious. Vascular surgeons have had to reinvent themselves due to traditional open vascular surgery drastically diminishing. Either that or they'd be out of a job.

The success of IR is manifold. Like much of radiology in the UK, there has been a 50% increase in IR procedures in the last decade. The sheer pace of technical development, the profusion of new techniques makes IR one of the fastest developing and most exciting specialities. Every week there is a new improvement, a new indication, a new bit of kit.

It is evolving so fast that IR is far out-stripping the evidence behind its use. Also anyone not paying attention to new developments gets left behind quickly. The techniques become almost too clever. As one interventionist said to me, 'We solve problems that clinicians don't know about in ways they don't understand. We cannulate vessels they don't know existed with a device they've never seen'.

Interventional radiology has changed the medical landscape in the last few decades. IR is seen as sexy and, naturally, every speciality wants a slice of the interventional pie. Particularly the surgical specialities that have had their practice turned on their head. The turf wars between IR and various other specialities are raging and will continue to rage and rage. Turf wars are occasionally ironic. For example, the chap (Moniz) who performed the first cerebral angiogram was a Portuguese neurosurgeon.

I can sit back and smile slightly as I am slightly removed from it. At the end of the day, it doesn't matter who delivers the service. It doesn't matter who is on the end of the needle, so long as they are well trained, well supported and delivering a good service. But turf wards must remain civil and constructive otherwise services suffer. And that is no good for our patients (see Rule #100).

The other aspect of this rule is not physical resistance but mental resistance from others. For example, you may confidently propose a specific action but others don't agree. If the others are assertive types, this can be a point-blank refusal with specific enunciation of the problem they have with your proposal. Or, if they are a bit more British, it may be a bit more of a passive protest, where they drag their heels, dawdle and dither until the thing doesn't happen through sheer inertia.

Either way, the clever interventional radiologist looks out for resistance from key individuals or the whole team. They actively listen for it. They have the ability to take stock and reassess. There is even a whole Human Factors jargon for this—'situational awareness'. What ever the problem is, they stop pushing. They reassess and, if it is in the best interests of the patient, they change their course of action.

The opposite is obstinacy. It is easy to understand how it develops. When someone has decided to do something high risk to a patient, they have to have self-belief and a singular focus. They want to do their best job. But add obstinacy to a degree of enthusiasm bordering on zeal then you have a dangerous combination. This gives rise to the joke, 'What's the difference between a interventional radiologist and a rhinoceros? One is thick-skinned, excitable and charges at everything. The other lives in Africa'.

The reason that experienced interventional radiologists are highly valued is not necessarily their slickness. Any numpty can become physically slick at any procedure. The older guys have a measured approach, their decision-making skills are honed. Decisions made before, during and after a procedure are what separates a slick chancer from a wise expert. Knowing precisely when to do something and when not to do something is the key. There are no short-cuts to this, it only comes with age, knowledge and experience (see Rule #28).

Chapter 23
Rule #23 / / Use Words Carefully

Clarity of communication is everything. A good test is ruined by a poor report. Never, ever write, "Clinical correlation advised". Ever.

—

Do your toes curl at the tautology 'CT scan'? Have you ever said, 'Where are the cows?' in response to the phrase 'lung fields?' Do your knuckles whiten whenever you read 'clinical correlation advised' in a radiology report? Do you secretly admire Channel 4's *Green Wing* radiologist character Dr Alan Statham?

Now read the following:

> They tend to obsess over the minutiae of subjects, and are prone to giving long detailed expositions, and the related corrections, and may gravitate to careers in academia or science where such obsessive attention to detail is often rewarded

You may be forgiven in thinking this is describing radiologist but it is actually describing the behaviour of those with Asperger's syndrome (or Higher Functioning Autism). Obsessive Compulsive Personality Disorder is also in part characterised by a form of pedantry with the correct following of rules, procedures and practices. As a result, pedantry is typically used negatively, as an insult, implying a personality defect.

The term 'pedant' comes from the Latin *paedagogare*, 'to teach', derived from Greek terms for 'child' and 'to lead'. So its roots are honourable. There are varying degrees of pedantry which is summarised well in Fowler's *Modern English Usage:*

> The term, then, is obviously a relative one: my pedantry is your scholarship, his reasonable accuracy, her irreducible minimum of education and someone else's ignorance.

I see nothing wrong with a degree of pedantry. Moreover, I am faintly proud of it. I do feel a bit embarrassed when it gets the better of me in a meeting or other public forum. A bit like wind, I suppose.

P. McCoubrie, *The Rules of Radiology*, https://doi.org/10.1007/978-3-030-65229-6_23

Radiologists inexorably become pedantic to some degree. It is partly due to our training and partly due to our working practices. Our tests are ranked by their ability to be specific and sensitive. Learning curves, ROC curves, operator dependencies are part of our working culture. We are always looking to be that bit better, that bit more accurate, that bit more specific. I therefore argue that we radiologists should embrace pedantry and be proud of doing so.

As the accuracy of our opinions is at the core of our very being, we are equally picky about the clarity of our formal reports. The written radiology report is the primary medium of a radiologist. Reports are a unique blend of art and science. The art is painting a vivid picture with words, the transcription of a greyscale image into a brief but lavish verbal pastiche. The science is the product of hypothetical-deductive reasoning, a probabilistic prediction of disease solely based on what we see.

Each radiologist has a unique reporting style. The structure, formatting, the choice of words and specific phrases makes it recognisably theirs. To a certain extent, the reports reflect the personality of the individual. The younger and more anxious the radiologist, the longer the report. The more idiosyncratic the radiologist, the more quirky the report. The more gregarious and extrovert the radiologist, the more amusing the report. And vice versa for all these.

Every single radiologist thinks their reports are the best. Their reports reflect their years of experience and considered expertise. They are proud of their output despite each one being very rarely ever seen or heard of again. I must admit a guilty secret of smiling whenever I see a report of mine from over a decade ago. It was a more innocent age back then when we took our time and savoured every syllable.

A radiologist feels a rosy glow when someone compliments them on their reports. There is a flicker of joy deep in their soul whenever they spot a trainee using one of 'their phrases'. Whereas if their reports come under criticism, the automatic reaction is defensive. An accusing finger pointing at a written report is a body blow for a radiologist. It takes a certain humility to add an addendum admitting that the original report was not in every way the very embodiment of absolute perfection.

Standardised reports or template reports haven't taken off in the UK to any great extent. Although embraced with gusto in certain parts of the world, the very mechanistic nature of these strips out any individual style. Plus most real-life template reports I've seen are detestably bland—tediously long things that I'd not want my name on the bottom of (see Rule #94).

An average radiologist produces thousands of reports a year. My reporting style is fairly concise; brevity being the soul of wit and all that. Some radiologists are damnably verbose, calling a spade a long-handled spatulous gardening implement. To them each picture is literally worth a thousand words. As we will see in Rule #24, a wordy report is usually a poor report.

Despite my relatively terse prose, I have calculated that I produce the equivalent of a PhD thesis every month. Which is an vast output, if you think about it. It is unmatched by virtually any other professional group. There is possibly one person in history who could match this—Dame Barbara Cartland—famed for writing over seven hundred books at the pace of six to seven thousand words a day. But then again, she dictated to a paid assistant and never had to wrestle with Voice Recognition (see Rule #86).

Given a radiologist's daily logorrhoea, the difficulty is maintaining a decent quality throughout. You need every report to be equally exemplary. It doesn't matter if you call it diligence, high professional standards, or pedantry. The argument is the same. Attention to detail indicates high professional standards. This is a self-evident goal that cannot be gainsaid.

But when is enough enough? Given the time pressures that radiologists are under then it could be argued that excessive attention to detail is a luxury that cannot be afforded. So it is a balance. Of course radiologists want to be proud of their reports but there is a mountain of work to get through. Other colleagues will be grinding their teeth if they see one of their brethren fart-arse around for twenty minutes as they craft the perfect conclusion.

I teach our registrars that the standard to aim for is a report that would cause no discomfort if read out in a court of law. Now that is a pretty high standard and it is usually a phrase that produces a palpable tension. But that is what must be produced. Corners cannot be cut (see Rule #90). A radiologist never knows when the nuances of one their reports will be absolutely crucial.

Just recently, I came across a small series of reports by a consultant radiologist that I didn't know. They were God-awful. Everything was wrong. They were inaccurate, poorly formatted and full of typos. The prose was in turn excessively long-winded (see Rule #24) then excessively terse (Rule #72) with some passages of exceptional rambling vagueness (Rule #29). They were so bad that a clinical colleague contacted me and said. "I've no idea what these reports mean: can you help interpret them?".

The problem with a poor report is that you cannot tell if this because the radiologist that wrote it is incompetent or if it is just a sloppy report from a competent radiologist. The end result is the same. A radiologist that is out of their depth will come across rambling, vague and inaccurate. But an expert radiologist can also come across rambling, vague and inaccurate, particularly if they rush. Which is, of course, why radiologists should never be tempted to do this, especially when exhorted to do so by clinicians (see Rule #52).

On the contrary, the best radiology reports are the product of a ordered brain that is assiduous in transcription of its workings. I've worked with some exceptional radiologists. One particular individual was so ordered, structured and methodical in their approach that he made difficult scans look incredibly self-evident. Another venerable radiologist delivered particularly eloquent radiological soliloquies, reports of such charm and suaveness, purring into the Dictaphone as if he was trying to entice it to bed.

This style can be mimicked but takes years to master. Meanwhile, young radiologists are taught basic rules for radiology reports. Always answer the clinical question, include pertinent negatives, avoid vague quantifiers, add a conclusion if the report is over four lines and so on and so forth. I would add two further absolute rules to be enforced with a rod of iron.

The first is 'Get off the fence (or explain why you are on it)' (more of which in Rule #29). The second is 'Never ever write 'Clinical Correlation Advised'. Ever'.

You may question my vehemence—why such vitriol over such an innocuous little phrase? The origin of this phrase is a rebuttal of poor quality clinical information. The joke being that the difference between most radiology requests and cereal boxes is that there is more clinically useful information on a cereal box.

Except, somewhere along the way, the use of 'clinical correlation advised' got distorted. Some sick individuals started randomly peppering reports with this phrase, apropos of nothing. For some it almost became a standard sign off. So it has lost any practical use. It has now become a joke phrase that is used by clinicians as a stick to beat us. It is for this reason that radiologists must swear to their favoured deity that they'll never use it, ever.

Chapter 24
Rule #24 / / Brevity Is King

The longer the report, the greater the uncertainty. Also, clinicians won't read it; anything longer than 4 lines and they skip to the conclusion.

—

When I was a younger radiologist I was proud of my detailed reports. I wanted clinicians to have both quality and quantity. I left nothing out; every organ was mentioned, all abnormal findings were included irrespective of their significance. Also, I wasn't afraid to show my workings. Not only did I detail the scan findings, but also included a brief exposition on my diagnostic reasoning and a differential diagnosis in light of the clinical details.

Textbook stuff, you might think. Surely this is what you expect of a radiology report. Documenting everything thoroughly, giving the clinician the unexpurgated truth. By leaving nothing out you are providing a safe and defensible report. Not that I would ever advocate defensive practice but being sued does prey on the mind these days.

I started to change my mind after an off-the-cuff and slightly awkward moment at an annual appraisal after I'd been a consultant for a few years. Midway through, and a apropos of nothing, my senior colleague tentatively said, 'Umm... your reports are a bit long'. Frowning at this minor slight, I politely retorted that I was proud of my work. I said that if a report happened to run several pages, it was because it was a complex case and I was just very thorough. She looked askance at me, cleared her throat, and never mentioned it again.

No one had said this before. I'd only ever received praise for my reports. This brief but earnest statement gnawed at me slightly over subsequent months. Was she right? Was I working under false assumptions? Had my ego got the better of me? (Correct answer—always yes). Being the thoughtful type, I began gazing at my navel (metaphorically).

At the same time (and for completely different reasons), I started a literature review of the evidence behind radiology reports. I couldn't help wondering what

P. McCoubrie, *The Rules of Radiology*, https://doi.org/10.1007/978-3-030-65229-6_24

had been written, what studies had been performed, what evidence lay behind what I and thousands of others spend our entire working lives doing. I was unprepared for what I found.

It emerged that, amongst other gems of wisdom, there was very good evidence that long reports are a Bad Thing. The longer the report, the more it was seen as uncertain. The literature was also littered with radiologists extolling brevity and giving countless ways in which to do this. Then, reading a single phrase in one paper (Martin, Can Assoc Radiol J, 1982) I had a revelatory moment. This read 'A report need not always be brief but it can always be concise'.

I saw the glaring error of my former verbose ways. How could I have been so foolish? I immediately began endeavouring for concision. Like an evangelical ex-smoker, I started proselytising. I probably annoyed my colleagues no end. I told all and sundry of my Damascene conversion to the As Concise As Possible way of thinking.

You might be thinking to yourself that this McCoubrie chap is a bit slow. A wise individual has always said less than necessary. This particular notion predates widespread literacy. For example there are several quotes from the Old Testament of the Bible that are around 2500 years old. For example Proverbs 17:28 (King James Version, 1604) reads, 'Even a fool, when he holds his peace, is counted wise: and he that shutteth his lips is esteemed a man of understanding'. Similar quotes can be found in Proverbs 15:2, Job 13:5 and Ecclesiastes 5:3.

When Shakespeare wrote *Hamlet* in around 1602, he coined the phrase, 'Brevity is the soul of wit'. The mistake is to think he was writing about humour, indicating that something succinct sounds wittier. He actually wrote this epigram for the vain and foolish character Polonius intending it to be used with a strong sense of irony. The word 'wit' at that time meant wisdom or acumen. Hence the phrase means 'the essence of wisdom is not talking too much'. The irony is that Polonius embarks on a self-contradictory windy speech denouncing the time wasted by rhetorical speeches. It's beautiful.

Now I know what you are thinking. You are thinking that this chapter is also laden with irony. It comprises several pages of rambling text about the need to be brief. And hahaha well done for spotting my cunning literary device. Except there is also ironically a lot to be said about being brief. Specifically that it isn't that easy.

In 1656, the French mathematician and philosopher Blaise Pascal wrote in a letter *'Je n'ai fait celle-ci plus longue que parce que je n'ai pas eu le loisir de la faire plus courte'*. This very roughly translates to 'I have made this longer than usual because I have not had time to make it shorter'. This witty excuse for the extravagant length of one of his letters was a memorable notion, particularly coming from one who was famed for imparting much in so few words.

This concept was new and fairly shocking. It was assimilated into the English language and became widespread. Variants of the same expression have been used by a number of luminaries over the last four centuries. Similar notions have also been expressed about giving speeches. In 1918, US President Woodrow Wilson was asked about the amount of time he spent preparing speeches to which he famously replied,

> It depends. If am I to speak for ten minutes, I need a week for preparation; if fifteen minutes, three days; if half an hour, two days; if an hour, I am ready now.

History therefore tells us that brevity is the treasured hallmark of a wise individual. Therefore concision in one's radiology reports is a worthy goal. But how, I hear you cry? There are plenty of authors who will tell you their opinions, much of it evidence-free guff. Fortunately I am here to sift the meagre wheat from the plentiful chaff. What follows is a pithy guide to succinctness.

There are two major methods of achieving the ideal laconic radiology report. The first is to omit findings. The second is to omit words. I should warn you that at this point, the science stops and the style starts. There is no single perfect method and good logical arguments for different approaches.

Omission of findings sounds horrifically risky but actually isn't. The way to do this is, first and foremost, answer the clinical question and then afterwards include pertinent negatives. Then stop. 'Pertinence' is the key motif as this is where your expertise comes in. A massive list of normal structures helps no one. It is truly useless. Resist the urge to pad out the report. Specifically avoid content-free sentences such as 'no other abnormality'.

For example, a normal cancer follow-up CT could read "(1) No locoregional recurrence (2) No metastatic disease (3) No new findings elsewhere". All said and done in 10 words. Job done. No point listing anything else. Radiologists who do this will be sought out and embraced by surgeons and oncologists alike.

Of course, that is an easy example. But radiologists make constant but deliberate choices to not mention certain findings. It comes with confidence and knowledge. A radiologist friend of mine nicely encapsulated this, 'There is a time in every radiologist's life when they stop mentioning simple renal cysts'. It is a truism. If you know the relevance of every finding, choosing what to exclude is actually straightforward.

Omitting words is paradoxically more tricky, more controversial and more difficult. There is no correct answer to the debate of full sentences *vs.* partial sentences. I omit verbs and definite articles for purposes of brevity. But I don't criticise colleagues that use full sentences for purposes of readability and to look more professional. I do criticise observational detachment—passive statements such as 'are seen', 'appears', 'note is made of'—they add absolutely nothing.

'Normal' is a report we've all seen many times. Some favour it's succinctness but falls flat as it doesn't answer the clinical question. Some reports mask their uncertainty by being brief, presumably on the assumption that what you don't say can't hurt you. This is fallacious. Concision should be considered and deliberate. It shouldn't be used as a way of hedging.

Beware extreme terseness. It makes difficult reading. I did hear of a radiologist who was fabled to have produced an X-ray report that read 'Bones. Sclerotic. Prostate'. I will grant you that it is extremely succinct but isn't immediately obvious that they think there is metastatic prostate cancer in the bones.

So how do we achieve this balance of readability and concision? It is through merciless expunging of extraneous words. Or as Kurt Langlotz has it, reducing 'a surfeit of superfluous and redundant pleonasms'. For example, there are famously twenty-eight ways to say 'normal'. Are you guilty of using 'no abnormality detected'?

Radiologists do inexplicably mangle the English language. Who the hell 'interrogates' the lungs? Omitting such words always helps readability and brevity. Reports are frequently littered with repetitive redundancy: interval change, mass lesion, total occlusion, close proximity, previous history. Such tautologies can be safely omitted too.

I do encourage radiologists to try the 'One paragraph challenge'. If you try really hard you can condense virtually every report. And if you do so regularly, clinicians might even read your reports properly. And they'll appreciate all the findings and all the nuance instead of skipping to the conclusion.

Chapter 25
Rule #25 / / Ditch The Stethoscope

Who are you trying to kid? You don't even know which one is 'lub' and which one is 'dub' anymore. Oh, and lose the bowtie. Seriously. It makes you look like a pillock.

—

Not long before I became a radiologist, I bought a new stethoscope, a new suit and a new pair of shoes. I was sitting a notoriously difficult postgraduate exam, the final part of the Membership of the Royal College of Physicians (MRCP). As it is a clinically-based exam, I needed to look like the part. One crucial aspect was to drape a recognisably expensive stethoscope around the back of your neck. This was the unspoken uniform for an aspiring physician. A lesser stethoscope just didn't cut the mustard.

I have a theory that postgraduate medical exams are largely a punishment devised by older and more bitter doctors, presumably because they feel that young doctors having far too easy a time of it. Part of my evidence is that these dratted exams are timed to have maximum disruptive impact on your life. This particular exam was in early July and so I spent most of my summer revising, bitterly missing out as others cavorted late into the long, warm evenings. And if anyone knows how to cavort, it is young doctors. Ah, those halcyon days of cavorting!

I actually had my radiology job already lined up but decided to sit the MRCP exam anyway. I was dithering as it was an expensive and time-consuming ordeal. Then a old and wise radiologist said to me 'If you don't [sit it], people will think you are a t**t', which sealed it. Suited and booted, I sat and passed the exam. Whether or not it was the thick rubber of my new stethoscope, my shiny new shoes or my clinical acumen, I'll never know.

Three months later I was a radiologist. I never wore a white coat again. I consigned the old guessing tubes to my bottom draw and haven't touched them since. In fact, it is so long since I used a stethoscope that I've forgotten which end goes in your mouth.

P. McCoubrie, *The Rules of Radiology*, https://doi.org/10.1007/978-3-030-65229-6_25

I was perplexed that a few consultant radiologists wore a white coat and still carried a stethoscope. This had me musing on the issue of visual identity amongst radiologists. How on earth do you recognise a radiologist? We don't have a uniform, we have no specific medical item that we all carry. Apart from a curious pale hue and stooped posture that comes from an indoor desk job with long hours, most radiologists just look like any other harried middle-aged person.

We in the UK have a particular nomenclature issue. We have radiographers and radiologists—two very similar words, related professions but quite different professional groups. In most countries, radiographers are known as 'X-ray techs'. UK Radiographers have a detailed three-year long degree-level training, whereas UK radiologists are medical qualified and have a minimum of twelve years of training.

There is no point railing against the UK status quo other than to point out that the similar words causes endless confusion and embarrassment. I was once at a formal function when a young female doctor draped her arm drunkenly around my shoulders and slurred into my ear 'You are my favourite radiographer'. I smiled woodenly, politely undraped her arm and excused myself.

And, of course, the general public has little perception of what radiologists or radiographers are. We lack a public image even though we are a reasonably large specialities that have been around for over 100 years. There are now more than twice as many radiologists as there are pathologists in the UK. Most radiologists have a short patter that they rattle off when someone asks them what kind of doctor they are. If you simply answer 'I'm a radiologist', you are inevitably met with a faint smile of ignorance.

I'm told that anaesthetists suffer the same problem. Everyone looks the same when dressed in scrubs. I'm told that this is why female anaesthetists tend to wear pearl necklaces. But the irony is that when the medical ordure hits the rotating ventilation device, everyone else panics and looks to the radiologists and the anaesthetists to help out. Surgeons are no longer the dominant heroic hospital speciality.

I've worked with many different radiologists and whilst most dress smartly (see Rule #87), each one has their own style. I've worked with radiologists that are shoe-obsessed and one that preferred to be barefoot. I know radiologists that dress like a scarecrow and some that would be at ease on a catwalk. Some radiologists always wear a suit and some aren't averse to a t-shirt. There is no one uniform approach, as it were.

There was a peculiar attack on neck ties in the UK in 2007. A rather evidence-free ban arose from a single publication from the Department of Health (or D'oh! as I like to call it). This concerned appropriate dress in the clinical environment to prevent the spread of infections, mainly the banning of the white coat, outlawing the tie and introducing the bare below the elbow rule.

A quick word about hospital-acquired infections. Obviously they are blot on the healthcare landscape, a stain on our glorious institutions. Reversing the trend of increasing infections caught in hospitals is vital for good patient care. This is the job of the Infection Control Team.

For those that don't know, Infection Control are the hospital equivalent of the Gestapo. Their edicts must be obeyed without question. Anyone seen to be stepping out of line incurs the full wrath of the Medical Director. White coats disappeared overnight as did wrist watches. Female colleagues had to remove treasured jewellery. My male colleagues had to stop wearing ties. I can't help thinking the plethora of open-collars makes the radiology department look like a louche firm of copywriters. Goodbye sartorial elegance, every day is now dress-down Friday.

Interestingly, the D'oh! proclamation had a subheading "Poor Practice" that stated, 'Ties are rarely laundered but worn daily. They perform no beneficial function in patient care and have been shown to be colonised by pathogens'. Unfortunately, these statements are all true. But you might argue that everything is everything is colonised by pathogens. Everything.

My main issue here is that the same document also states, 'It is good practice to dress in a manner which is likely to inspire public confidence", as "general appearance [is a] proxy measure of competence'. Bit of a dichotomy, eh? Do you want a professional looking doctor or a potentially cleaner doctor? Sadly, we know the answer already.

One particular conspiracy theory cannot be ignored. This is the emasculation theory. This centres on the shape of the tie, plus the way it unsubtly points towards the nether regions. Hence a woolly blunted-ended tie can be seen as a direct statement of masculinity, or lack of it. It therefore follows that forcible removal of the tie altogether is tantamount to castration. I don't really buy it myself but it is food for thought.

The other aspect is the tie as a social statement. The selection of tie states membership of a certain club, or perhaps, that one is worryingly keen on cartoon characters. There is also the issue of exerting the nuances of one's personality. Just this morning on the way into work as I was idly flicking traces of black pudding and absinthe from my Royal College tie, I wondered what messages I was giving out.

The loss of ties and white coats is deeply ironic. Neck attire and the white coat arose as part protective clothing and part evidence of cleanliness. The rest of the world have discarded neither ties nor white coats. Yet they are not seized with doctor's clothing related-infection control hysteria. In fact, outside the UK, the white coat remains a global doctors uniform.

Men could get round the tie issue by adopting bow ties. However, a professor at my alma mater used to say that wearing a bow tie marked one out as a pillock. Even though I know many fine gentlemen who besport bow ties, I can't shake his words from my head. Cravat, anyone?

So, faced with an official proscription of ties, why not embrace this emancipation? Who honestly really likes the physical discomfort of wearing a tie anyway? Surely we will all mellow slightly as an indirect result. Despite this liberality, I still feel slightly underdressed and paradoxically uncomfortable.

Alternatively, partly in demonstration, you could radically change your professional garb. Many wear scrubs these days. Some places have colour-coded scrubs, so you can tell a heavily tattooed and hefty porter from a heavily tattooed and hefty surgeon. You could chose the logical extreme. The *reductio ad absurdum* is to perform all one's professional duties dressed in the way least likely to transmit infection; lightly oiled and wearing only a swimming costume.

Fundamentally, professional garb boils down to professional identity. What you wear in the workplace is your badge of office. For some, the white coat is part of it. For others, Lannaec's (or Leared's) acoustic aid is akin to an ID badge. For me, the bigger your badge of office, the more it indicates your insecurity. If your clothing is all about projecting an image, I'd say you are trying too hard. Making power statements with an ostentatious apparel doesn't mark as a person as 'above the fray', it marks them as 'an inadequate'.

Chapter 26
Rule #26 / / CT Is Easy

Real hardcore radiologists do loads and loads of plain radiographs (NB they are not counting - see Rule #12). They do them quickly but take pride only in their accuracy. Anyone who 'doesn't do plain films anymore' is a work-shy fop.

—

Friday the 8th of November 1895 was particularly momentous. It was on this date that the medical speciality of diagnostic radiology was born. On that special day, a fifty year old Professor of Physics at the University of Würzburg, Wilhelm Conrad Röntgen, was experimenting with vacuum tubes and first documented X-rays. It just goes to show that a man left alone in a dark room messing around with electronic gadgets can occasionally achieve something worthwhile.

Two weeks later, Frau Anna Röntgen famously exclaimed, 'I have seen my death' when her husband took the now famous X-ray picture of her hand. He published his original paper 'On A New Kind Of Rays' (Über eine neue Art von Strahlen) on 28th December in the same year. Clearly journal reviewers were a lot slicker back then.

As vacuum tube technology was relatively widespread, the development of medical X-rays was rapid. Within a month of the announcement, several medical radiographs had been made in Europe and the US. By June 1896, X-rays were being used by battlefield surgeons to locate bullets. Pioneering trauma surgeons were also probably blaming early proto-radiologists for their sluggish service and poor quality images.

The 8th of November is now World Radiology Day, an appropriate tribute for a modest and reticent man. Showered with honours, Röntgen won the first Nobel Prize for Physics in 1901 and donated the prize money to his University department. He refused to patent any of his technology, wanting society as a whole to benefit. Which is pretty amazing. Most academics are not well off. If offered 150 782 Swedish Kroner (~$1 m) as a prize, many would at least buy themselves new leather elbow patches for their tweed jacket.

P. McCoubrie, *The Rules of Radiology*, https://doi.org/10.1007/978-3-030-65229-6_26

For the next sixty years, the X-ray was all we had. Whether you called them roentgenograms, skiagrams or plain radiographs, silver-impregnated X-ray film ruled for a century. The radiologists of the day initially had nothing else. But they soon discovered how to pimp their X-rays. They added contrast. Various dense (or lucent) substances were added to the body to make specific structures show up more clearly.

Each contrast innovation was an advance but my radiological forefathers didn't half invent some barbaric contrast studies. Barium sulphate poured up the derrière seems like a walk in the part compared to pneumoencephalography. And barium wasn't the worst contrast agent. In fact, iodinated poppy seed oil injected into various body cavities pales into insignificance next to Thorotrast. Thorotrast was a great contrast agent, by all accounts. Downside is that thorium is kind of pretty radioactive. The worst bit is that they knew.

Irrespective of this one-step forward, two-steps back story of contrast studies, the X-ray was always there. And it is still here. My department does nearly a thousand X-rays a day. We do around 4–5% more each year, year on year. It is bizarre, if you think about it. A century-old technology still growing more popular. Although the UK population is ageing, we aren't getting 4–5% sicker every year. And it isn't an unmet need; we've offered a same-day service for over 2 decades.

My personal theories on the growth of plain radiographs are, as you might expect, slightly controversial. I think a little bit of it is defensive medicine, clinicians covering their own backside without a decent reason. A little bit of it is change in medical practice, where radiographs are slowly becoming more an inseparable part of medical practice. But I think the majority of this growth is that clinicians increasingly feel that doing nothing isn't an option.

Faced with a patient in distress, clinicians feel they should do something (see Rule #16). Sometimes this is an unthinking knee-jerk. For example, faced with someone with chest pain, a chest radiograph must therefore follow. More often this is akin to placebo therapy, it won't help you as a doctor but the patient may get some reassurance. Your aching knee might feel better now that the X-ray has shown it isn't fractured. It was never fractured, no one in their right mind thought it was. But somehow an X-ray helps.

Given this daily deluge of radiographs across the world, most of which are normal or near normal, someone needs to look at them. The purist would say that a radiologist should report them all. It is the Gold Standard. The purist would also say that they should be 'hot reported', fed directly to a radiologist the moment the image is available, irrespective of the time of day.

I have no problem with this Gold Standard of health care. It'd be fantastic, quite literally so; a utter fantasy. Quite unaffordable on a population basis. You'd need an army of radiologists available 24/7, purposively slightly under-employed so as to have immediate availability. Virtually no country can afford that.

At the other end of the spectrum, you have no radiologists. In some very low income countries the public hospitals have no radiologists or at best, intermittent and partial cover. The person looking at the X-ray is the person who asked for it.

In the UK, matters have changed in the last twenty years. We have slipped spectacularly from Gold Standard to Bog Standard. Back then, most hospitals had most of the X-rays formally reported by a radiologist. Some managed to look at 100%, some less. Most consultant radiologists were reporting somewhere between 5000 and 40,000 radiographs a year.

Now it is a different story. Most hospitals have stopped reporting every single last radiograph. Certain x-rays are just not reported at all. Patients in fracture clinic get their x-rays looked at then and there. A later formal report is neither wanted nor needed. This makes sense, to be quite honest. But some go unreported for the simple reason of understaffing. Some hospitals have such a shortage that their radiologists do no plain film reporting.

I have absolutely no problem with non-radiologists reporting X-rays. So long as they are well trained, well supported, working to high standards and take responsibility for their actions, they can be very valued members of the department.

But there are two problems with this. First, there is a big shortages of other health care professionals and other medical specialities, some more so than the UK's 35% shortage of radiologists. It makes no sense to divert these staff groups to fill the reporting void. Second, if standards of training and practice are not of a similar standard to that provided by a radiologist, you are condoning a second class service.

One issue that complicates matters is that UK radiologists are only too happy to give up reporting the plain radiographs. I've seen it many times. They don't drop CT or MRI but, given the chance, the plain radiographs are dropped like a stone. Or at least reported as a lower priority, after the CT and MRI.

I've embarrassingly witnessed myself doing this. Faced with a monumental pile of work, I found myself leaving the radiographs to last. Or worst, dodging them altogether, hoping someone else will pick them up. Why is this? What underlies this behaviour?

Given that a modern CT comprises several thousand images, it seems counterintuitive to favour this over one or two images. So it isn't that. Another explanation is that CT and MRI have higher status and reporting them brings kudos. But I don't buy that either. No one looks at your output stats and rank those that do more CT accordingly.

My explanation is simple. Plain radiographs are just harder then CT. Specifically, plain radiographs are harder to get right. They are more subtle and nuanced—the sensitivity and specificity is lower. You have to work harder to be accurate. You really have to concentrate more. Reporting a big pile of radiographs is mentally taxing.

This explains the maxim of why 'all radiologists become a plain film radiologist eventually'. It isn't that younger radiologists are bad at reporting plain radiographs, it is just that it takes years to get slick at it. It explains why radiologists in their late career are worth their weight in gold, motoring effortlessly through mountains of plain radiographs, whilst younger colleagues creep haltingly through a much smaller number of studies.

CT is truly easier. The sensitivity and specificity is higher. Despite the complexity of visual images, diagnoses are easier to make on CT and, to a lesser extent, MRI. So favouring CT is actually slothful. But it is one thing to favour CT but another thing altogether to refuse to report plain films.

Excuses for not reporting plain films such as 'lack of time', 'they are boring/too easy' are bogus. Derogation from plain radiograph reporting should be explicitly recognised as unacceptable. It should be called out as an antisocial act, a bone fide sign of radiological turpitude.

On the up side, plain film reporting should be celebrated and promoted as the intellectual challenge it truly is. I can see it now. 'Join Club Rad—report a radiograph today'. Or even 'Make Radiographs Great Again'?

Chapter 27
Rule #27 / / Don't Answer The Phone

It is not for you. The more you answer the phone, the more it rings. Even if it is for you, it isn't a social call. Ignoring it encourages face-to-face consultations. These are better for clinical care and certainly a lot more fun for the radiologist.

—

When I was a fresh-faced house officer, face-to-face conversations with a radiologist were the only type of interaction possible. If you wanted anything other than a plain radiograph, it needed discussion. Your request would languish in the 'routine' tray until you spoke to a radiologist. So if you wanted your inpatient CT this month, you needed to speak to a radiologist.

Raising a radiologist on the phone wasn't a starter. They were busy people who did not simply drop what they were doing to speak to a clinician. It was nothing personal, just the way it was. If you wanted to speak to a radiologist, you had to go and find one.

The first step was to navigate around the back rooms of the radiology department. Most radiology departments had grown over decades without any planning all, sprawling around the hospital like a drunk octopus. It wasn't deliberately done to confuse interlopers, just haphazard multiple phases of building.

Consequently, once you stepped away from the waiting room, you discovered a veritable maze. I spent hours wandering down vaguely familiar but increasingly dark and small corridors. At one stage I considered spooling a reel of string behind me, as I plunged into the bowels of the radiology department, half expecting a Minotaur at it's heart (Fig. 27.1).

Finding a radiologist twenty-five years ago held further hazards. Stumble across the wrong one and you'd get either screamed at by one of the psychopaths or given the third degree by the sneering ones. You knew which ones were reasonable, in which part of the labyrinth they hung out and the style they liked.

Some were three-sentence types. You had five seconds to blurt out a maximum of three terse sentences before they lost focus and started to walk off. If you didn't

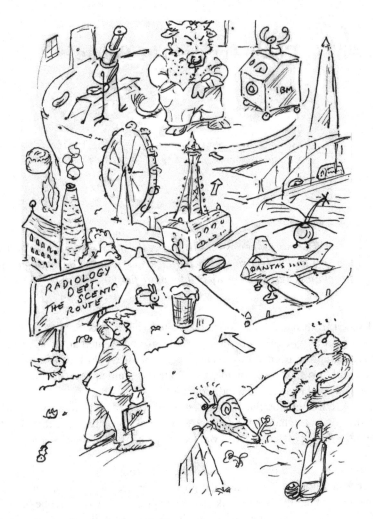

Fig. 27.1 Half expecting a minotaur at its' heart

have the request card in their hand within the first three seconds, all was lost. They generally rarely stopped moving; you had to talk as you sidled along.

Some were clearly lonely and bored, they kicked out a chair when you walked in and wanted to know everything. As you started your spiel, they closed their eyes, arched their fingers and flopped their head back, ready to hear your thesis about the patient. The end of your entreaty was ritualistic. You briefly summarising the patient's case details and why such-and-such a procedure was indicated. This then either elicited a smile and a nod or a shake of the head whilst they held the door open.

This system was clearly very radiologist-centric: they were in control and you had to dance to their tune. But as a junior doctor, once you knew the ropes, it worked fairly slickly. You got to know most of the normal radiologists and steered clear of the bonkers ones. You knew how to address them and once they got to know you, it was all very straightforward.

The down side was the shoe leather. In a big hospital, the radiology department could be several minutes walk away. As a junior doctor I once worked on a medical unit five floors above the radiology department in a building with very sluggish lifts. After six months there, I was whippet-thin and had thighs of steel. The brogues needed new soles and heels twice that year.

And, of course, time. I didn't mind; I knew I wanted to be a radiologist. But for others, it was a chore. Schlepping to the radiology department several times a day takes out a decent chunk of your working day; time you can ill afford when you are very busy.

The main thing, in fact, 90% of the deal from the radiologists point of view, was that you got to look the relevant junior doctor in the eye, establish that there was no ...erm... bovine excrement involved. If you are a radiologist, you know how much BS comes our way. If you aren't a radiologist, well, we get a lot. The time to filter this out is at the discussion or vetting stage (see Rules #53 and #67).

Another 5% is clarity of communication through a face-to-face discussion. That way, the radiologist can focus the scan on the correct organs and do it in a timely manner. If the patient is sick, you do it now: clear the scanner and get the patient in next. If they are not so sick, it can be done at a time of mutual convenience.

The other 5% is a discursive or educational role. The more complex the case, the more important it is to run it past someone else, if only to make sure they agree. The more junior the doctor, the more educational this discussion is. Radiologists can turn a dull clerical task of organising a scan into a positive educational experience (see Rule #55).

Of course, the majority of scans don't need in-depth discussion. Hauling your carcass across the hospital to discuss every scan is utterly unnecessary. And given the sheer numbers of scans being done every day, the hospital would grind to a halt if this was the case.

I have a concept of a hierarchy of communication; a three-layer pyramid, if you like. The top layer is face-to-face discussion: highly effective and nuanced, allowing verbal and non-verbal communication. But we simply don't have time (see Rule #43) so we have to ration this for urgent, complex or nuanced cases. Hence the pyramid has a narrow peak.

The bottom layer is written communication, the large flat base of the pyramid. A succinct written request form is adequate for most circumstances. Although time-efficient for all concerned, it has marked limitations. It is a largely one-way transaction; no interaction is possible. Space is limited, hence detail is impossible.

There is also no time guarantee; you write it and send it off hoping for the best, it can sit there for an indefinite time. Forms can (and do) get lost, physically or in the electronic ether. There have been many scandals where, for various nefarious reasons, scores of years-old request cards have been found simply stuffed in drawers. Hence written communication is the poor cousin, the lowest rung of the ladder.

The middle layer of the pyramid is telephonic communication. This 140 year-old method is still relevant. It is highly time-efficient, particularly with mobile technologies. It allows immediate communication over near-infinite distance. So, you might ask, given the clear pragmatic advantages, why I am exhorting radiologists to ignore ringing phones?

Clearly if it is for you, you should answer it. This can be a problem. Some radiologists never do. They are like deaf and blind eels. They notoriously fail to engage with written and telephonic communication, wriggling free of any commitment. Whether this is a self-protection in a hyper-contactable world or just laziness, I don't know. Irrespective, it is poor practice and indefensible.

Most often the phone call isn't for you. And because radiologists make very expensive receptionists, you shouldn't answer it. This isn't arrogance, it is pragmatism. However, there are three bigger reasons not to answer the phone.

First, the immediacy is all one-way. It is great for the person making the call but highly disruptive for the other person. The shrill ringing is explicitly designed to be difficult to ignore. Few radiologists can easily drop what they are doing with no impact. We don't just sit around waiting for the phone to ring. And being disturbed whilst you looking at a scan is a sure way to miss things. No one wants to encourage errors.

The second reason is grasping the difference between efficiency and effectiveness. Sure, the phone is efficient but it isn't a terribly effective means of communication. A small proportion of communication *in toto* is the words we use, estimated at less than 10%. Non-verbal communication is everything. Tone of voice and body language are 90% of the deal.

The third reason, the meta-reason, if you like, is that it encourages poor systems of work. I work at a hospital where the emergency department was specifically designed to have a radiologist immediately next door, 24/7. Yet still clinicians ring from just 20 m away. And this is the rub. Face-to-face discussion should be promoted and encouraged, not supplanted by the telephone.

The crucial issue is deliberately and specifically choosing what is fine on a request card (or electronic equivalent), what is appropriate to phone about and what should be discussed face-to-face. Fortunately the answer is easy. And I can provide it to you right here and now.

My mantra on this is simple. The sicker the patient, the more complex the patient, the more I want to discuss it face-to-face. If they are neither sick nor complex, just a standard request card is fine. And only ring me if you are not physically in the hospital or have lost the use of your legs.

Chapter 28
Rule #28 / / Stay Safe The Easy Way

In a high-risk patient, the lowest rate of complications occurs when you don't meddle. Contrast nephropathy is unheard of if you don't give contrast. Patients don't exsanguinate from a biopsy that didn't happen.

—

Primum non nocere is Latin for 'first, do no harm'. It is a premium bit of bioethics. Also known as non-maleficence, all doctors learn it, usually early in their student career. The second top concept, 'do good' (beneficence) is not so prominent. There is a fine line, I find, between wise ethical advice and stating the bleeding obvious.

'Do good' is bit too obvious an instruction for a doctor isn't it? Fine advice, perhaps, if you are a company with high ethical standards (cf. Google's now-dropped unofficial motto 'Don't be evil'). But the raison d'être of medical practice is to help the ill. Only a stark-raving psychopath would think otherwise. Sadly, we do have a few with psychopathic tendencies in our ranks but even they wouldn't deviate from being generally beneficial.

'First, do no harm' is quite odd, if you think about it. Why are we told this very specific negative and almost equally self-evident concept? The logical progression of this would include a massive list of specific negative instructions including perhaps 'don't lick the patients' and 'no running side bets on resuscitation attempts'.

You'll have some people tell you that *primum non nocere* it is part of the Hippocratic Oath (it isn't) that all graduating doctors recite (we don't). Two glaring errors: Hippocrates was Greek and also he never said or wrote this. He did have a segment in his *Epidemics* which is similar. Very roughly translated from the original Greek it means 'try to help your patients when you can, and when you can't, at least try not to make things worse'.

It is fairly sensible stuff and makes you want to read a little more of the writings of our medical forefather from Kos. Similarly enthused, I bought a translation of the Hippocratic corpus many years ago, eager to learn from the oldest of

P. McCoubrie, *The Rules of Radiology*, https://doi.org/10.1007/978-3-030-65229-6_28

medical teachers. I did learn one key message: don't bother. I found the rest of his writing to be largely utter mumbo-jumbo.

The phrase *primum non nocere* sounds ancient but certainly is not. Depending on which authority you believe, it was either coined by Thomas Sydenham in the late 1600s, a French pathologist (Chomel) in the early 1800s or variety of US authors around 1860. It is true that anything said in Latin sounds more weighty and profound. For example, '*Podex perfectus es*' sounds very classy but is, in fact, a crude insult (I'll give you a clue - *podex* = the anal region).

Medicine has a long history of appropriating Latin and/or Greek words to name things or invent new jargon. We've been at it for centuries. Sometimes it is odd— the *acetabulum* or hip socket is Latin for 'vinegar cup'. Sometimes it is beautiful such as 'proctalgia fugax' meaning 'transient pain in the backside' (*n.b.* it's a medical condition, not an insult). Sometimes it is a gratuitous insult such as 'lignoce-phalic' a hybrid of the Latin for 'wood' and Greek for 'of the head'.

There are those who see a sinister side to these ethical mantras. They believe 'first, do no harm' is being used as a stick to beat us. It can be interpreted as meaning that harm of any kind is derogation of duty of care, irrespective of the intention of the original action. This fuels malpractice action which in turn fuels intense risk aversion and fuels defensive medicine where the premier motto is 'first, cover your own backside'.

If you take 'first, do no harm' to a logical extreme, it would emasculate every physician as virtually no test or treatment is totally risk free. If the main logical goal of medicine is the absolute avoidance of harm at all costs, then surgeons would be out of business. Radiologists may have to shut up shop too, perhaps offering only ultrasound (it being the only truly 100% safe scanning modality). Medical practice would become a nihilistic enterprise, focussed on prognostication and shrugs. But homeopathy would thrive. Clearly if that happens, the whole idea has major flaws.

The problem is that there are many people at this end of the spectrum. They have unrealistic expectations of perfection in healthcare. For them, negative health outcomes are not 'just one of those things'. If treatment doesn't work perfectly, perhaps there has been idiosyncratic side effects or unforeseen complications, then someone must have done something wrong, someone must be to blame. It is based on ignorance and very destructive. It makes the doctor:patient relationship rather fraught.

You would have thought that modern medical practice is so good that we'd be able to predict which patients might not do so well. You might imagine that the wealth of research would it easy to prediction who won't benefit from certain therapies. You would be excused in believing that doctors could accurately estimate who is likely to suffer side effects or complications but no, our estimates are vague and imprecise.

We are getting better at this, slowly. Real life risk–benefit decisions are difficult to make. Estimates are inaccurate, particularly as applicable to the individual patient. One can talk in general terms about probabilities in certain populations but rarely with certainty about one person. And prognostication is both difficult and inaccurate over even short periods of time. Mapping out someones health journey over twenty fours is hard enough, never mind what is likely to happen over the next week or month.

Discussion about risk–benefit is fraught with difficulties. The evidence is often presented in detailed statistics. But statistical concepts are confusing and often counter-intuitive. Your average patient is, in the nicest possible way, statistically illiterate. And to make this worse your average doctor is inept at communicating the complexities of this. To make it even worse, unconscious bias is always lurking under the surface in both the minds of the doctor and patient.

Daniel Kahneman, in his Magnus Opus 'Thinking, Fast and Slow', details a number of these biases. Generally, he says, people overestimate the probability of unlikely events and this colours their decision making. This is particularly true if they are vivid risks, such as their leg dropping off. People can be affect by how data is presented. A 0.0001% risk of harm sounds much better than 1 in 100,000, doesn't it? Yet is ten times as bad. A 'disease that kills 1286 out of 10,000' sounds much worse that 'a disease with 24.14% mortality', yet is half as lethal.

To give a radiological example, let us consider the radiation dose from a standard CT of the abdomen and pelvis. Official figures say this type of scan gives the individual an estimated lifetime risk of fatal cancer of 1 in 2000. This sounds horrendous. But 1 in 3 in the UK die of cancer anyway. So it increases your risk from 0.33 to 0.3305. Which doesn't sound so bad.

This isn't to denigrate the risk of harm from ionising radiation, which we take seriously (see Rule #13). Radiation is intrinsic to X-ray, CT and nuclear medicine techniques. Risk-benefit arguments apply to every one of these tests. Although MRI can kill you with flying oxygen cylinders, rip metal splinters from your eye, stop your pacemaker, burn your skin and wipe your credit cards, it is completely safe. Ultrasound is totally safe. Getting on and off the couch is more hazardous than the scan itself.

Interventional radiology is much safer than open, laparoscopic or endoscopic surgery. That is one of it's main appeals. But it most certainly isn't risk free, particularly when you are dealing with rather small yet crucial structures or attempting something heroic and possibly lifesaving.

Everything has side effects. Life has risk. I would never ride a motorbike or horse and would only climb a ladder under duress. The reason is simple: I regularly scan those who fall off and it isn't pretty. Medical practice is similar fraught with complex risks, many of which are unpredictable. As a result iatrogenic illness is only a breath away. It is potentially everywhere and we have to be alert to it.

Radiologists, as I have shown, are equally affected by bias. We should neither overestimate our capacity to help nor underestimate our capacity to cause harm. And yet we should deal with risk appropriately. Systems that are intended to prevent harm can hinder in equal measure.

The crux of this Rule rests on the largely optional nature of radiology. Although radiology is at the heart of modern medical practice, good quality medical practice can still exist without it. Sure, radiology makes modern medicine easier and better but if someone cannot have a particular test or procedure, there are ways around this. Safe alternatives exist.

Sometimes doing nothing is the best thing, the safest thing. You may be faced with a high risk patient, either from frailty, co-existent illnesses or dementia. An adverse dalliance with a radiologist is probably the last thing that they need. Don't be that person to tip them over the edge. Stay safe the easy way.

Chapter 29
Rule #29 / / Get Off The Fence

*Do not let the fear of being wrong rob you of the joy of being right. If you abso-
lutely have to equivocate, you are only allowed one hedge per sentence, "There
appears to be a possible nodule" tells much, yet almost nothing.*

—

Over the last twenty years I've read a lot of other radiologist's reports. These are
mainly those of my colleagues as part of local discussions but I've seen reports
from all over the world. The majority are functional and dry technical affairs. They
are factual but immemorable. They get the job done without fuss.

Occasionally you'll come across a real cracker, a report that makes you stop
and smile. Radiologists develop an eye for such things, a bit like a surgeon who
appreciates a neatly sutured wound or a builder that admires precisely laid brick-
work. Not only have I developed great respect for a good report but I've ruminated
on how to emulate the reports of my radiological role models.

After more than a decade of introspection and combing the literature on the
subject, the key ingredients turn out to be fairly simple. Succinctness is mandatory; a verbose report will never be a great report (see Rule #24). A great report
must be accurate, which is where expertise comes in. Accuracy is rarely accidental; you have to really know your onions (see Rule #39). When brevity and accuracy are combined with the third ingredient, clarity, then you have the building
blocks of something special.

I've worked with some radiologists whose reports are sublime. If you watch
them in action, they churn out beautiful reports quite effortlessly, not a hair out
of place, not a bead of sweat, not a ounce of strain evident on their fizzog. It is a
product of years of experience, years of deliberate practice, years of honing their
trade.

I freely admit my jealousy. It takes me considerable effort to turn out a report
of which I am truly proud. I don't mind this purely on the basis that one should be
prepared to suffer for one's art. There is a saying that a piece of poetry or prose

© The Author(s), under exclusive license to Springer Nature Switzerland AG 2021   113
P. McCoubrie, *The Rules of Radiology*, https://doi.org/10.1007/978-3-030-65229-6_29

produced without effort is rarely worth reading. Some go so far as to insist that something worth reading should have half-killed its author.

Half-killing might be pushing it a bit. No radiologist wants to stagger home from work, steaming from the ears, mentally wounded by their daily reporting effort. And after all, there are no plaudits for quality of reports, only the sheer number produced (see Rule #12).

I get a tingle up my spine when watching a great radiologist who is also a peerless communicator. It is the pinnacle of performance, a thing of beauty to be marvelled at, something to treasured. Each of their reports are like perfectly cut diamonds; flawless and shining, irrespective of the angle at which you hold them up for inspection.

On the flip side, some reports induce heart-sink. I often find myself huffing and softly cursing as I wade through the turgid outpourings of some radiologists. I shake my head and sigh dramatically at the obtuse observations. When faced with a multi-page report with at least one hedge in every sentence, I am almost impressed at its unhelpfulness.

When I say hedge, I'm talking about quite unnecessary vagueness when a clear diagnosis can be made. The commonest form is the inclusion of vague quantifiers such as 'probable', 'possible', 'may represent', 'suspicious' and so on (the list is endless). For example, 'there is a possible pneumothorax' is a seriously opaque statement. Of course, sometimes diagnostic uncertainty exists and has to be articulated. But there is never an excuse for saying something 'cannot be excluded' (see Rule #33).

Radiologists have been called the modern soothsayers. There is some truth to this analogy. We sift through the entrails, look for signs and then make pronouncements, some of which are quite baffling. I would love to put out something like this:

CT abdomen with contrast
I count the grains of sand on the beach and measure the sea; I understand the speech of
the dumb and hear the voiceless; I read the pattern woven in the very fabric of man.
Comment: entrails are auspicious

This notwithstanding, most radiologists want their reports to be less abstruse than the predictions of the Delphic Oracle. There are, however, a few who seem to be channelling the Pythia herself. Every observation is couched in ambiguity. Little is concrete, all is doubt. Every finding is riddled with further questions. Furious mental dithering makes their reports are as substantial as fog.

Radiologists have a bad name for being ambiguous. The badge of our speciality is said to be 'A weasel eating a waffle under a hedge'. I'm not clear what drives hedging. There are several reasons I can think of. Sometimes it is an inadvertent bad habit; sometimes it is a mistaken belief that hedging is good practice. Sometimes it represents a lack of self-belief; sometimes it is covering up for ignorance. Whatever the reason, hedging is indefensible.

There is balance, of course. I've met radiologists who would not dream of equivocating. To these monochrome radiologists greyscale doesn't exist. Doubt is for wimps. They like it sharp and snappy. Their differential diagnosis rarely reaches two conditions. The problem is that life isn't like that. These radiologists are never in doubt but seldom correct.

So how can radiologists achieve a balance on this? Well, the key is to avoid unnecessary and excessive hedging. Here are few tips. As stated above you are only allowed one hedge per sentence. Let us consider the choice phrase of 'No focal active lung lesion'. It is impressive, actually. To fit three hedges into a five word sentence takes some doing. Firstly, although there may be nothing 'focal' what about something diffuse? And, secondly, what the hell does 'active' actually mean? Answer—nothing; it is utterly meaningless in radiology. Lastly, 'lesion' is both a hedge and a tautology of focal—ever heard of a non-focal lesion? Quite.

Radiologists are renowned for mangling the English language. Since when did it become OK to summarise a normal CT pulmonary angiogram as 'Negative for pulmonary embolus'? Why is the word 'no' suddenly not good enough? And why do we describe things like joint spaces and alignment of joints as 'preserved'? They've never been salted or pickled. Terms like this are imprecise, vague and hence should be resisted.

'Appears' is a loathsome but widespread hedge term. As in 'There appears to be a rib fracture'. Why 'appears'? Either there is or there isn't. It seems to stem from an erroneous belief that if you are wrong, the hedge protects you as you only said 'appears'. But of course, it doesn't. You just add a layer of uncertainty when you should be doing the exact opposite.

The same argument is true about 'evidence of'. It is a hedge and a grossly overused one at that. Specifically, it is wrongly used when describing something that can seen directly. When looking at an X-ray of a ruddy great carving knife sticking out of someone's skull, you don't write 'there is evidence of a carving knife sticking out of the skull'. Whereas some things cannot be directly observed. You cannot see a concept or syndrome. So 'there is evidence of assault' would be correct.

I have come up with a term called the 'dangling hedge'. This is where you state an ambiguous finding and then just leave it there, dangling in the breeze. For example, 'There is a possible cystic lesion in the pancreas' is stated and then is never mentioned again. No attempt is made to explain its significance, hazard a guess at it's nature or give guidance on the next most appropriate management steps. It is particularly poor reporting practice.

The word 'significant' is also a poor word. You can use it if both you and the clinician have precisely the same definition of significance. Given that this is pretty rare, you'd be wise to avoid it. Its main use is as a hedge. 'No significant lymphadenopathy' is a common howler. When I see it, I ask, 'What is insignificant lymphadenopathy?'. It doesn't exist, of course. Ipso facto neither does significant lymphadenopathy.

Once you've chosen to express yourself with clarity then you must pay attention to correct grammar, punctuation, and formatting. Some favour structured reports, others favour prose. However you do it, structure in reports is a Good Thing (see Rule #94). Clear organisation of ideas into ordered paragraphs lays bare your diagnostic thinking. Be sure to deal with the important issues early in the report otherwise major findings can get lost in the text.

Demanding clarity in radiology reports isn't a pedantic issue. Vague reports can be dangerous. The medico-legal literature (particularly that of Leonard Berlin) is strewn with examples where vagueness or ambiguity led the clinician to inappropriate management, sometimes leading to death of the patient.

I can simply summarise how to avoiding hedging as 'Get off the fence. If you can't then (i) explain why you are on it and (ii) how you propose to get off it'. You would have thought this is both fairly clear and fairly simple. But sadly it is far from universal practice. So, until that time, my work on this planet is not yet done.

Chapter 30
Rule #30 / / Don't Pick Fights

Arguing with clinicians is like wrestling with a pig in mud...after a while you real-
ise the pig likes it.

—

Imagine yourself having had a frontal lobotomy. Or the next closest thing for those of a certain age, a heavy lunch washed down with a few glasses of wine. Got it? OK. Now visualise yourself in this serene and imperturbable state. Picture yourself in this state working as a radiologist, beaming beatifically at all and sundry; the very picture of saintly benevolence.

A clinician arrives to discuss a patient. The dialogue starts benignly but a chain of events leads to deterioration of the tone. Despite the initial positive mood your smile fades and your calmness cracks. Mental thunderclouds start to gather. The conversation lurches from constructive to destructive. The consultation descends into argument.

A short time later, having failed to reconcile anything, both parties part company, thoroughly annoyed and cursing one another. The poor patient at the centre of the argument has had their care advanced not one iota. In fact, it has hit a speed bump. Hopefully this ding-dong hasn't upset things, somehow hindering their health journey.

I should admit that full blown arguments in the workplace aren't that common for radiologists. I don't want to over-egg the pudding. The majority of interactions are perfectly civil. Even when the radiologist and the clinician profoundly disagree about something, the large proportion of interactions remain cordial. It is only after the door is firmly closed that each party heaps scorn on everything the other one said or did.

Sometimes it is the radiologist who is at fault. Even the calmest radiologists can lose their composure (see Rule #3). Instead of forgiveness and understanding (see Rule #8), they seize upon any perceived slight. They know they shouldn't but they do. It is hard not to. We don't all have the patience of Job. When you are on

P. McCoubrie, *The Rules of Radiology*, https://doi.org/10.1007/978-3-030-65229-6_30

the sharp end of yet another jibe from some smart-arse clinician, they are lucky they don't get their head slammed in the door, never mind receive a mild verbal rebuke.

I've known some particularly argumentative radiologists. You know the sort, the ones that could start an argument in an empty room. The ones that have no filter and blurt out all manner of offensive guff. The ones that get complaints by the dozen and eventually are sent to mandatory anger-management classes.

Sometimes the radiologist is blameless. Radiologists do encounter aggressive clinicians quite frequently, a scenario sufficiently common that it deserves a Rule all of its own (Rule #38). Not wanting to be too picky but I'd like to distinguish aggression from assertiveness. Assertiveness is fine. In fact, it is to be encouraged. An assertive person lays out precisely what they want and why they want it. There is no waffle. It is very time efficient and like a breath of fresh air.

I've worked with some particularly intelligent clinicians who revel in the cut and thrust of academe. They welcome a bit of verbal sparring, a chance to unsheathe the mental rapier and duel with a like-minded intellect. It may start as light and frothy banter but they hate to lose a point of principle. Such discussions can therefore get heated and rather passionate, particularly if you have the clinician on the metaphorical ropes. But the key issue is that the tone remains civil throughout. Ultimately, such discussions are an enjoyable and benign intellectual work-out.

But some clinicians are just habitually rude. They are unthinking boors. They have no charm, no class, no warmth, no wit, no subtlety, no humility, and no grace. Whilst they might be laughable figures, they never say anything even faintly amusing. Their idea of a joke is a crass comment, an illiterate insult, a casual act of cruelty.

Some might see this bullishness and lack of complexity as refreshingly upfront. I don't. At all. These people are bullies. And I hate bullies. There are unspoken rules of basic decency in Britain. We don't punch down; we don't kick the vulnerable or voiceless. Whereas these churlish individuals always aim below the belt and prefer to kick those who are down.

From an anthropological point of view, radiologists are not in the higher echelons. Radiology is not a macho speciality. Ethnographically, radiology ranks fairly low in the medical pecking order. Therefore the loutish and domineering clinician sees radiologists as beneath them in a very real sense. Hence radiologists are fair game for a bit of aggressive subjugation.

Despite the thick skin that radiologists have, criticism and insults still sting, even from an acknowledged medical hooligan. It is difficult not to retaliate. But if you do counter-attack, you are descending to their level. Going head-to-head in an attempt to prove that you are right never works. It is highly destructive to both individuals.

People can be offensive without intending it. Take, for example, discrimination. I once worked with a female radiologist who looked a few decades younger than she was. She told me horrible tales of causal sexism. She was regularly patronised by male clinicians, they sprawled on her reporting desk, they chatted her up in the workplace, she was ogled and objectified, had her job 'mansplained' to her and much more. I felt ill as she recounted these tales.

Similarly, my colleagues with different skin colour, different cultural heritage, and different sexuality can all tell tales of discrimination. They tell me that some of it is overt, some of it is subtle and some of it is institutionalised. I find this intensely disappointing. Dammit, we are supposed to be living in a supposedly-civilised country. No doubt things are better than the gratuitous excesses of the past but we've still got a way to go.

Which is where this rule comes in. It is an exhortation not to engage with disreputable critics. As a concept or saying, advice about not wrestling with pigs is as old as the hills. The Bible says 'Answer not a fool according to his folly, lest thou also be like unto him' (Proverbs 26:4). Similar phrases have been passed down as folk wisdom ever since.

The boorish clinician is the Pig in this analogy. They are someone whose beliefs are formulaically fortified against self-doubt. Stereotypically, this is a surgeon. There is a cartoon of a surgical brain that is mapped out as 75% ego, 24.5% scalpel skills and the remaining 0.5% is tiny area called 'the nucleus of self-doubt'. But Piggishness isn't exclusive to surgeons. I've been metaphorically charged at by hog-like anaesthetists and porcine physicians.

The analogy is worthy of exploring. Pigs are adept at avoiding being pinned down. Pigs have cloven hooves which give them superior traction in the mire. Pigs do not mind getting dirty one bit. More specifically, the Pig is happy to see everyone else down in the mud. This means that others have to stoop to adopt their tactics. Therefore the Pig doesn't even have to win. Because their opponents debase themselves by entering the mire, the Pig benefits from the struggle irrespective of the outcome.

Attempting to argue with a pig-headed clinician turns a civilised discussion into a no-holds barred fight, where each party lashes out, demeans and insults others. Rather than encouraging contrition and self-improvement by admitting that you could possibly be wrong, you tear down the other to assert that they are worse than you.

These are the precise moments when you have a choice. You can choose to enter the mud pit and wrestle with the pig. Don't: merely re-read Rule #3. Or you take a deep breath, collect yourself and find clarity. Align your actions with your highest intentions. Imagine the type of person, the type of doctor, the type of radiologist you want to be. And read Rule #38.

As an intellectual exercise, you can spot a conversation that is turning a little sour, a clinical encounter that is becoming a little porcine. When a clinician starts to employ logical fallacies, they are revealing their trotters and curly tail. Take, for example, the Strawman gambit. In this common tactic, the clinician misrepresents your argument to make it easier to attack. It is a weak and dirty argument but when employed with skill and aplomb, it can be most effective.

The good news is that if you are aware of such logical fallacies, you can easily brush them aside. You know, for example, that if someone employs an *ad hominem* attack then they have not a single decent point worth making. Personal attacks carry no weight and can be safely ignored.

Criticism can be constructive if fair. But be careful in accepting all criticism at face-value. Don't take criticism from someone you don't respect. If you wouldn't seek advice from a particular person, don't accept criticism from them. Their opinions are of little worth. Ignore them.

Prevention of a fight is better than mopping up afterwards. Try not to go anywhere near any clinical arena that resembles a farmyard. If a clinician looks like a Pig, smells like a Pig and acts like a Pig then they are a Pig. Be like a duck. Float along the river effortlessly, enjoy the scenery and gentle flow of the water. Let the cruel words wash over you and drain off safely. Don't get into arguments with clinicians as the wasted energy means that the radiologist always comes off worse. Meanwhile the patient suffers whilst you are squabbling.

Chapter 31
Rule #31 / / Beware The 'Good' Case

The impressive case that you think you've nailed and thus triumphantly show to all and sundry is only a biopsy away from being a classic mistake.

___

Before 2006 when English radiology went digital *en masse*, I had steadily amassed a goodly collection of interesting cases on x-ray film. Two large cardboard boxes in my office contained a large selection that I'd copied and squirrelled away over the previous 7 years. Ostensibly they were for teaching but some were purely for personal fascination.

I had examples of some highly unusual conditions. Sometimes it was because they were conditions of historical interest; I had a great Thorotrast spleen CT (see Rule #26). Sometimes it was because I'd been there and watched a case unfold; a series of linked studies told a graphic patient story. Sometimes the cases were mistakes that I'd made; or even better, mistakes of colleagues that I'd picked up. Sometimes it was purely for the amusement factor; every radiologist is contractually obliged to have a radiograph of an improbably large household object lodged in the rectum.

Some radiologists are obsessive. They systemically collect vast numbers of cases and rigorously categorise them, like a butterfly collector. These individuals become infamous for their encyclopaedic film collection. But therein lies a deep irony. Their fanaticism is only equally by a singular lack of enthusiasm over sharing the fruits of their labours. Few are allowed to glimpse the collection, even fewer could actually touch their amassed cases. The number of people who learn anything from this hoard are minimal.

My film collection was well used, ragged at the edges and mildly chaotic. Bit like me, really. Except I'm not covered in sticky fingerprints and traces of chinagraph pencil. Well, not usually. My half-decent collection would be sought out by trainees for teaching. It was my films they wanted to see; I was reduced to a bystander.

P. McCoubrie, *The Rules of Radiology*, https://doi.org/10.1007/978-3-030-65229-6_31

Without a decent collection of radiographs, a radiologist has to stoop to some lower medium, something inferior, like PowerPoint. And they'd have to show images stolen from the internet. Trying to teach with someone else's images is curiously unsatisfactory. It's OK initially but later on proves to be ultimately false and hollow. A bit like accidentally drinking alcohol-free beer. Or worse, decaffeinated coffee (see Rule #70).

With a decent box of teaching films and a lightbox then you were good for several hours. The hot-seat style of teaching has been a staple of radiological education for several decades. If done well it can be curiously effective. If done badly it can be an instrument of mass humiliation.

I made the mistake of loaning out cases for colleagues to use for teaching. I never saw a single one of them again. My prize rabbits - gone! My beautiful chest radiograph of Holt-Oram syndrome was stolen by a radiologist who is now dead. I should add that the radiologist in question was very much alive when they borrowed it. And perhaps I should also add that their demise was nothing to do with a missing teaching film. I'm not that vindictive.

I learnt my lesson. Shakespeare wrote 'Neither a borrower or a lender be' and the Bard had it about right. I can quite understand it. If a colleague slid you a cardboard film packet containing an exquisite teaching case, the temptation to palm it into your collection afterwards was almost irresistible. I never did but the issue with physical film was that once it was gone, it was gone. You rarely kept a separate record of the case details.

Acquiring a good case for your collection back then just involved copying the original, taking care to mask the name of the patient off. Or printing an anonymised copy if it was digitally acquired. Obviously the modern world of radiology is digital. Now you would have thought this would make all these many issues just evaporate. You just simply copy the digital file and everyone is happy, no? Theoretically, yes. But the reality is a little different and surprisingly complicated.

Yes, single images can be exported easily as standard graphics files such as JPEG. But that doesn't work for CT and MRI which have hundreds of images. The global native file format used in digital radiology is a specific file format called DICOM. I don't want to get too boringly technical but DICOM files are quite complex. Each file contains not only the image data but also several hundred items of metadata, including about thirty items of unique forms of patient ID.

So, if you want to build a library of teaching cases that you can take outside the hospital, you have to export the images and strip out all every single bit of patient ID. Obviously the images have to be totally and utterly anonymous. Anonymity in a teaching case is a *sine qua non*. In the UK, we have very strict data laws about this. Most countries have similar data protection legislation that keeps radiologists on their toes about digital anonymity.

I can confirm that digital anonymisation is much more hassle than it sounds. You have to use a specific bit of software that not only reads DICOM images but also allows editing of the metadata. 99% of commercial software can't do this. At the time of writing, the market leader is a bit of software called Osirix, which only runs on Apple Computers. Hence if you go to a radiology conference, you might think they are all Mac fanboys. But no. They merely have to have a MacBook Pro to maintain a teaching library.

To be honest, I hanker for the days of a lightbox and x-ray films. It was so easy. Organising a teaching session merely involved grabbing a handful of film packets and off you went. No need for a laptop, charger, cables and having to rely on a gloomy VGA projector turning your beautiful files into a blurry on-screen grey mush.

The plus side was that film packets could be used for other things. I must admit that I used an empty cardboard one as a professional prop. If you were seen talking empty-handed in a corridor then this could be interpreted by the boss as Idling. Not so if you had a film packet in your hand. A film packet indicated Purpose. Even if the film packet only contained a well thumbed copy of a salacious periodical and an empty pie wrapper.

For all this nostalgia, my film collection is gone. It got sent for digitisation and irretrievably lost. I'll spare you the details, mainly as the woeful tale of incompetence really boils my piss. So I've had to start from scratch, building a fresh digital teaching library. Which in some ways is refreshing but in others utterly annoying.

A mistake I was keen to not replicate is adding cases to your teaching collection without somehow affirming that you had the right diagnosis. Or at least ensuring that the case was from sufficiently far away or a sufficiently long time ago that no one can gainsay you.

This rule explicitly looks at this ultimate pratfall where a proudly presented classic case turns out to be a classic mistake. I've done this several times. I proudly diagnosed a chordoma which later turn out to be nothing of the sort (see Rule #47). I've been so sure of my diagnostic accuracy that I offered to eat my pants if I was wrong (and I should have - I was - see Rule #40).

It is an easy cognitive trap for anyone to fall in. When the clinical history is *so* convincing. The radiological findings are *almost* pathognomic. You've been seeking to make this particular diagnosis for *years*. All the stars line up and boom! You are flat on your intellectual backside with metaphorical custard pie all over your face.

What actually happens is that you overly trust your gut feelings. Your intuition tells you all you need to know. Your inner chimp shouts so loudly and it is so proud of itself that it cannot hear the forebrain urging caution. Hence you wave your new and exciting case at your colleagues—the professional equivalent of beating your chest and whooping loudly. Which makes the subsequent ignominy even worse.

It isn't that you weren't aware that you could be wrong. You were perfectly aware of other conditions on the differential diagnosis. It is just you discounted them prematurely. Sometimes you discounted them through ignorance. It is understandable. Everyone has gaps in their knowledge. Sometimes you discounted them due to rarity. But faulty statistical reasoning is almost universal. Plus there are so many rare conditions that there is always at least one of them in the hospital (see Rule #52). But mainly you discounted other diagnoses through allowing Type 1 thinking to dominate (see Rule #20).

The common cognitive flaw that underlies this pitfall also tells you the answer. Don't bray about exciting cases until the diagnostic dust has settled. Wait for confirmation. Wait for the biopsy. Wait for the MRI to complement the CT. You still get to look clever, you still get to share your diagnostic triumph and there is far less likelihood of looking like an ass.

Chapter 32
Rule #32 / / Don't Fret About Complications

If you haven't encountered complications during a procedure, you haven't done enough of them. They will still happen irrespective of preparation, training, skill, carefulness and clinical likelihood. The complications you worry about don't happen and the ones that do are unforeseeable (see Rule #5).

———

I was a young student when I discovered that things could go wrong in medicine. Of course, I was vaguely aware of this but it wasn't something I had given due attention. My innocent twenty-one year old brain thought that complications were the reward for sloppiness or incompetence. Complications simply didn't happen to assiduous and competent doctors.

The heads of medical students are stuffed full of touchingly naive ideals. They are exhorted to be the next generation of healers. They are told that their every deed, thought and action can have a therapeutic benefit. They are pumped full of shiny principles and dazzled with science as the medical world unfurls around them. The future of medicine is painted so bright that they need sunglasses. Such is their sense of wonder and marvel that some of them get caught up in the hubris of it all.

These poor deluded youngsters believe that medical practice is a benign hi-tech utopia. It is a soft-focussed Elysian idyll. All illness is diagnosable, all investigations benign, all symptoms ameliorable, and all treatments successful. Furthermore they believe that the doctor lies at the heart of it all, a kind of sainted conductor of the healthcare orchestra.

This vision is markedly at odds with reality, which they soon discover as they begin their clinical career. I remember the heady days of buying a stethoscope and casually slinging it into the posterior cervical position for the first time. But as the students tread the wards for the first time you see them falter and blink with cognitive dissonance. They fail to recognise the low-tech dystopia around them. The sharp-focus reality hits them hard between the eyes.

P. McCoubrie, *The Rules of Radiology*, https://doi.org/10.1007/978-3-030-65229-6_32

The mirage of a medical Shangri-La evaporates. It turns out that real medicine is imprecise, messy and occasionally quite unbearably smelly. Diagnosis is fleeting and uncertain, investigations are far from benign. Symptom control is difficult; there certainly isn't a perfect pill for every ill. Furthermore when you lift the lid on the healthcare machine you find that doctors are mere medium-sized cogs.

Anyway, this rule is not a diatribe on the state of medical education. It is all about risk and understanding of it. Risk is part of life and most people think they understand it. But as we saw in Rule #28, our understanding of risk is riddled with bias. There is plenty of evidence that doctors are just as prone to flawed thinking about risk as the general population.

Certainly healthcare used to be much more risky. Attitudes to complications once verged on the blasé. There was a documented operation with a uniquely high complication rate. In pre-anaesthetic days the speed of the surgeon was a virtue. The surgeon in question (Robert Liston) was famously able to amputate a leg in twenty-eight seconds. The story goes that such was his haste to amputate a patient's leg, that he cut off the fingers of his surgical assistant. The patient sadly succumbed later of gangrene as did the wounded assistant. Not only that but an on-looker keeled over dead at the barbaric sight. It is the only recorded operation to have a 300% mortality rate.

This surgical recklessness has never really existed in radiology. I don't know of a single radiologist who is known as 'Slasher' or anything remotely similar. We are a largely conservative bunch (with a small 'c'). We balk at the idea of iatrogenic complications. Most radiologists choose the easy way to avoid complications—we pass on the opportunity (see Rule #28). You see, those of us who are ham-fisted tend not to wield needles and other sharp objects in the workplace. There is choice over the matter. Dabblers are dangerous. If you are doing something potentially dangerous, you should be slick at it or not be doing it at all. Training is, of course, different. That needs supervision.

I heard of an apocryphal tale of a poor radiology registrar who was asked to do a liver biopsy but was too afraid to admit they'd not done one before. It seemed to go well. Tissue was obtained and placed in the specimen pot. But the pathology report came back 'Normal chest wall, normal pleura, normal lung, normal pleura, normal kidney, normal colon. This is not a liver biopsy; this is a kebab'.

Doctors hate complications because, in their mind, complications are the sole preserve of a substandard doctor. Radiologists generally see themselves as above average (despite this being a statistical impossibility). When a radiologist causes a complication then they cannot shake the feeling that they are a bad doctor. They know it isn't true but it is only human to feel this way.

Famed neurosurgeon, Henry Marsh, writes very movingly about this in his first book *Do no harm*, baring his soul about operations that went wrong. And when things go wrong in the brain, they have the potential to go very, very wrong. Another surgeon with a gift for taut prose is Atul Gawande. His 2002 book *Complications* is a masterpiece. It highlights that decision-making at the clinical coal-face is very difficult and, essentially, how doctors will never always get it right. Read both books, I urge you. I've not spoiled the plot of either.

The absolute key to this Rule is the fact that doctors don't always get it right. This happens less often in the best hospitals, with the best medical teams, with the latest tech, with the slickest processes. But it still happens. The human body is complex in ways we don't yet understand. Disease is fickle, occasionally difficult to detect and unpredictable in its course. Treatment success is rarely guaranteed: what works for one doesn't always work for another.

There is also statistical inevitability. If you do something often enough then the rare and unusual will eventually happen. For example, we radiologists get through barrel-loads of water-soluble iodinated contrast media every year. I'm not kidding. Around twenty litres a day at our place. It is pretty innocuous stuff and we slosh it around in a relatively wanton manner. Serious reactions to intravenous contrast happen very rarely, probably less than 1 in 50 000. Damned rare. But if you do 50 000 scans a year then, on average, a serious reaction will occur annually.

A good radiology department will be prepared for this. Rare and serious complications should be planned for just as much as the commoner but less worrying complications. There should be protocols about managing the complication. Staff should be trained to deal with them. Suitable facilities and equipment should be nearby. This is so that when you fail, you should fail safely (see Rule #35).

Despite slickness to the n-th degree, routine procedures still lead to injury or even death. It is unthinkable but sometimes it just happens. In these instances there is no particular rhyme or reason. I know several radiologists that wish they had a time machine. They would love to replay a particular day but approach it quite differently. This is the day when despite all their skill, all their training, things went unexpectedly and horribly wrong.

For many years the approach to dealing with complications was profoundly unhelpful. Individuals didn't talk openly about it. At best, there'd be a hand on the shoulder and 'never mind, old chap'. But iatrogenic injury was fundamentally seen as your fault. You did it. No one else was to blame. At worst, it'd be dismissed as 'one of things'. That anything went wrong was strenuously denied. For centuries those suffering fatal complications were literally buried.

Denial of complications is utter madness. Despite the irrefutable arguments against it, I can cite many examples of just this. It isn't just individuals. Whole organisations are often involved. Some would argue institutions seek protect their reputation with a destructive ferocity, much more than individuals can or would do. But it happens again and again.

This approach stifles any positive outcomes. No important learning points can be extracted. No lessons can be taught to others. The lack of free discussion denies any therapeutic conversations; feelings are bottled up and sleep is lost. The closing of medical ranks alienates surviving patients and their families. The lack of apology or explanation accentuates anger and grief.

Therefore the only logical way forward is frank honesty. Don't deny or play down complications. Of course you try to prevent them at source through good practice. But state them simply and unapologetically. Don't worry about them. Have a system for dealing with them but don't be hampered by your fear of them.

In addition to honesty, implement a constant drive to reduce them. Acknowledge them, record them, analyse them and try to learn from them (see Rule #51). As we will review in Rule #93, look at what went wrong, rather than who was wrong. But in the meanwhile, don't worry about potential complications. Worrying is thinking gone toxic. It can paralyse skilled individuals. Focus on the task in hand. Focus on the patient in front of you. Give them 100% of your attention and deal with complications as and when they arise.

Chapter 33
Rule #33 / / We Are Not In The Business Of Exclusion

No test is 100% sensitive. We don't do 'rule outs'. Ever.

—

Professor Sir Howard Middlemiss was a radiological giant of his time. Although he died over 30 years ago, his memory lives on. I would have loved to have met him but sadly he was before my time. I heard a quote of his that firmly places him in my pantheon of Radiological Gods. It was said that he wanted a sign put up in the reception area of his radiology department that said, "We are not in the business of exclusion ".

This adage could equally be a rallying cry for twenty-first century radiologists. Particularly if you have high clinical standards and loathe sloppiness of medical thought, word and deed. Specifically, if you believe that sloppiness of deed stems from sloppiness of word, which in turn derives from sloppiness of thought.

When I was a newly appointed consultant, the terms 'Rule out x' or 'Exclude y' on a radiology request used to be infrequent and minor irritations. Now every second request contains now bears these poisonous words. Like a buzzing mosquito they tick all the three qualities for being annoying: (1) noxious but not physically harmful; (2) unpredictable and intermittent; (3) persistent but of uncertain origin.

It is an affectation. It is a trend. I understand that. You'd have thought that I would have become habituated. You'd have thought that I would be able to rise above it. Well, I've tried. I've adopted mindfulness techniques and breathing exercises. Yet it still annoys the bejesus out of me.

So I asked clinicians why they write this. They always state, "Well obviously I didn't mean that". So I reply, "Why did you put it then?". To which they look at the floor, walls and ceiling whilst saying 'erm' a lot. The other thing that I cannot let pass is when clinicians are asking for a scan by delivering a minor medical monologue and then ruin it by finishing with "So we'd like to *rule out* a hepatorhubarboma, please". To which I cannot help but clap my hands and say "Ooooh, you were doing so well until the end!".

I suspect the aetiology of this verbal pandemic is the pernicious effect of US medical culture spilling across the Atlantic. After all *Grey's Anatomy, House* and *ER* make up a significant proportion of the unofficial British medical curriculum. UK medical dramas have relatively little impact. We simply cannot match the Hollywood glamour. US audiences get a suave George Clooney playing the flamboyant Dr Doug Ross in *ER*; we get the stolid Derek Thompson playing mild-mannered Charlie Fairhead in *Casualty* for over 30 years.

Most UK medics in the maelstrom of a medical emergency would love to be able to shout out 'I want a FBC and Chem-7, stat!'. Even though no-one says 'stat' on this side of the pond. And we aren't quite sure what a 'Chem-7' is either. Furthermore, being British, we'd not shout it but ask politely. Or just get on with it ourselves, quietly. You can therefore understand how Brits are now aping their apparently sexier transatlantic cousins when they ask for everything to be 'excluded' or 'ruled out'.

Some of my colleagues frown at my frustration, puzzled at clumps of hair that I've just torn out (again). Indeed you may be wondering why I am getting all het up. Is 'exclusion' or 'ruling out' such a medical sin? Well, yes, it is abominable. It isn't pedantry, honestly. Let me explain.

First up, it is an anathema to high standards of medical practice. It spurns the laudable goal of diagnostic acumen; diagnostic indecision is embraced 'just in case'. It raises a louche middle finger at knowledge-based expertise; who needs clinical expertise when you have scanners to tell you the answer? It blatantly ignores the 'clinical method'—probabilistic hypothetico-deductive reasoning—based on history taking and clinical examination. It purposively rejects the model on which medical practice of the last two centuries has been built on.

Rather than using carefully selected investigations to confirm a diagnosis (sometimes called a 'Rule-in'), investigations are used broadly, frequently and in a semi-random fashion. But the bizarre thinking is the negative investigational paradigm. A 'rule-out' is performed explicitly hoping for a normal scan. It is like discharging a shotgun into the night sky to confirm no birds are flying past. It is illogical and indefensible as well as clinically and morally lazy.

Second, it reveals ignorance on behalf of the clinician. Now I am no guru of clinical epidemiology. Quite the reverse. I've always found medical statistics textbooks a reliable cure for insomnia. But ask a junior doctor about Bayesian reasoning and nine out of ten of them fish-mouth quite predictably. I remind them that virtually no radiological test is 100% sensitive and specific so I cannot 'rule out' anything, ever. They then blink at me like I am talking Greek. Occasionally there is a glimmer of recognition when I mention pre- and post-test probabilities. Not often, though.

Third, such language influences thoughts. I hear otherwise sensible doctors say things like, 'Well the CT excluded a hepatorhubarboma'. To which I cannot help but say, 'No, the CT is normal but it doesn't *exclude* a hepatorhubarboma'. Clinicians develop inappropriate dependence on and faith in test results. This is not necessarily true in an older generation of doctor who grew up without the luxuries of 24/7 scanners on tap. But the younger generation are much more reliant. Some are so hidebound that they seem unable to break wind without a CT to confirm the presence of rectal gas.

Fourth, it is wasteful. Inadequate triage leads to high negative rates and cost inefficiency. For example, a local audit of 1000 consecutive CT urograms showed the pick up rate for transitional cell tumours was just three percent. Similarly, twenty-five percent of scans looking for pulmonary emboli were positive a decade ago. It felt like a worthy and interesting thing to do. Now the pick up rate is in single figures. Normal pulmonary arteries were once a rare and fascinating structure but the sheer volume of the blighters has rendered them distinctly mundane. Finding a significant thrombus these days brings the registrars running to gawp.

Lastly, and most importantly, 'ruling out' is bad for patients. It is not that patients like having tests (they don't). Nor is it that tests are risky (they most certainly can be). It isn't even the diagnostic delay or personal inconvenience that multiple investigations bring. It is that the doctor:patient relationship is betrayed. Inappropriately extensive investigation can be disguised and sold to the patient as thorough and hence caring medicine. The truth is that the doctor is transferring risk to the patient under the guise of being thorough. 'Ruling out' is defensive medicine, plain and simple.

A lot of words have been written about defensive medicine. Oddly some have sought to justify their increasingly defensive practice, arguing it isn't a bad thing. Some have accepted it isn't ideal but have put finger to keyboard to explain their actions. As you might imagine, I have firm opinions on defensive medicine. I feel that it is a cancer eating away at key healthcare relationships. It turns the doctor:patient relationship into a lie. The guiding principle of defensive practice is not doing the best for the patient but first and foremost protecting yourself against litigation and complaints. And then kidding yourself that the patient is your first concern.

It turns the radiologist:clinician relationship into a farce. The discussions about scans are nothing to do with appropriateness and performing targeting investigations. The defensive clinician is quite happy to lie freely about the patient to the radiologist, exaggerating or even inventing symptoms purely to get the investigation done. The goal of investigation in the defensive model is not to help the patient but to cover the doctor's arse. Except I am not a pair of underpants. I will not cover anyone's backside.

I'm not blaming the individual clinician for all this reprehensible behaviour. It isn't their fault. Well, it is. But they are simply responding to societal change. You might imagine that we are in a modern world full of enlightened thought. You might feel that most people recognise that modern medicine is 'VUCA' —volatile, uncertain, complex and ambiguous. You might also hope that people don't seek to blame an individual when things go wrong but rather look why the system failed. But you'd be wrong on all three counts.

To practice radiology in today's environment is to have the spectre of litigation and the demon of complaints (Fig. 33.1) sat on either shoulder as you work. Well,

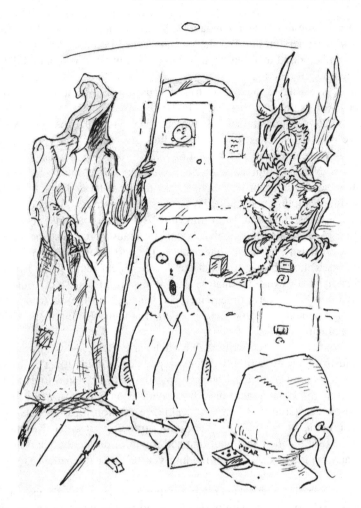

Fig. 33.1 The spectre of litigation and the demon of complaints

it isn't, actually. It is that you imagine that they are there. Everyone talks about them so much that you imagine that litigation and complaints are commonplace. Newspapers inflate any medical misdemeanour into a full-blown scandal. The truth of the matter is that successful litigation and serious complaints are becoming more common but still relatively rare. The average UK radiologist has little to worry about.

We should reject defensive practice, 'rule outs' and simply stick to good quality medical practice, based on the clinical method. The first step of which is to listen to the patient. They will tell you what they are worried about. If they then complain because you ignored that, then you only have yourself to blame.

Chapter 34
Rule #34 / / Trust Your Clinical Instincts

Take a brief history and tailor the examination appropriately—the patient is trying to tell you their diagnosis. However, if your barium enema patient starts Cheyne-Stokes breathing just as you are seeing the caecum properly, you should probably stop.

___

When I was a young radiologist I performed hundreds and hundreds of barium enemas. It was how you cut your radiological teeth in those days. Mainly because radiology, like any other trade, delegates the least pleasant parts of the job to the most junior. However, like any keen newbie, I threw myself into the task at hand.

Barium enemas are very easy in theory. Tube up the bum, run in some barium, take a few pictures, job done. However they are very easy to do badly. It is also very easy to cause considerable discomfort for the patient. Consequently there is a certain pride in achieving a good quality study where the patient will still look you in the eye afterwards. The gold standard is that they not only look you in the eye but say a genuine 'thank you' afterward.

In the odd Proustian moment I think back to those happy and innocent times, nostalgically musing *'ou sont les enemas d'antan'*? I can smell the faint reek of burnt plastic as I sealed my 100 mm cut film (yes, I am that old). I can hear the tutting of the radiographer as my size fourteens trod on the screening pedal for far too long (yes, I have enormous feet).

The other 99% of the time I'm just glad that barium enemas have been superseded by CT colonoscopy (CTC). I can confirm that CTCs are a million times easier for both staff and patient alike. Admittedly I am yet to be on the receiving end of a rectal tube but I've been on the giving end many hundreds of times. To date no one has fainted, sworn or sobbed during one of my CTCs. If only I could say the same about my barium enema patients.

The one constant feature between a barium enema and a CTC is the cup of NHS tea given as a restorative afterwards. NHS tea is a curious culinary

P. McCoubrie, *The Rules of Radiology*, https://doi.org/10.1007/978-3-030-65229-6_34

phenomena, somehow tasteless yet unpleasant. Being the curious sort, I opened an NHS tea bag once. It seemed to contain a blend of volcanic dust, pencil shavings and mouse droppings. Which might explain a few things.

Anyway. This Rule concerns procedural protocols and when to deviate from them. Every single radiological procedure has a correct way of being done. Sometimes these are purely an oral description, sometimes they are a massive standard operating protocol. My institution has both. It depends on a number of factors.

Writing a protocol for, say, the correct procedure for locating one's own buttocks may be slight overkill. Having said that I know certain individuals that have difficulty finding their backside with both hands and a map. But for a complex new technique, a protocol is damned good idea. An example is our CTC protocol written when we launched with an off-site service in 2014. Now in its ninth version, it spans forty-four pages and makes life very easy.

Any radiological procedure has a standard protocol. Sometimes this is utterly invariant. For example, a PA chest radiograph is ninety-nine percent the same the world over. There is one way of doing it. It has been in the textbooks for decades and no one has found a better way of doing it.

The newer and more complex the procedure, the more it will vary. Every radiologist and every institution across the world will believe that their way of doing it is the best. Not only that but the debates around protocol and technique are a massive, massive thing in radiology. If you aren't a radiologist, you wouldn't believe how much time and effort goes into this. If you are a radiologist, this will be depressingly familiar.

The radiology journals are full of articles detailing an alleged improvement to an existing technique. Authors present variable amounts of evidence of varying quality to support their argument. But as we saw in Rule #17, these studies are often small, retrospective and riddled with bias. Interestingly this type of article outnumbers articles describing new procedures by a thousand to one.

As a result I can almost guarantee that if you search for evidence behind variations in technique, you'll find conflicting advice. One paper might say that injections of flobblob-globulin help improve image quality and decrease side effects. Yet another seemingly identical study pooh-poohs its use as a singularly dangerous and expensive manoeuvre.

This results in mass confusion. Hard data about how to improve procedures get lost amidst the background noise. On a backdrop of this disarray, there can be only one true victor. This is the consensus paper. Ostensibly this is a good idea. When faced with scant evidence, the opinions of the great and good are the next best thing. The collated views of a bunch of experts saves us mere mortals an awful lot of time and effort.

I've seen consensus papers done very well. If you use an formal consensus method you are onto a winner. If you combine this with a highly formulaic method of combing the scientific literature for evidence then you usually produce something worthwhile. Formalised consensus methods avoid bias by design. I have some form here. Many moons ago I wrote a 23 000-word Masters thesis describing a large Delphi study.

I've also seen consensus papers done very badly. I've seen a bullish professor present their so-called evidence at a conference and then cajole their mates to ratify this as a position statement, thereby justifying their dubious practices. I've seen experts have massive fallouts over precise wording and who should be first author and so forth, leading to irreconcilable rifts.

A decent standards document or consensus paper can be worth its weight in gold, truly pushing up quality standards through harmonisation. It helps to have a bit of a stick to complement this paper carrot. This stick usually takes the format of some kind of mandatory audit with an unsubtle threat to those who aren't up to scratch.

On the flip side, a badly done consensus paper helps no-one. They usually set unachievable standards such as 24/7 provision of something that most hospitals struggle to provide for eight hours a day, five days a week. Or they are overtly protectionist, recommending that people exactly like the authors should be the only ones allowed to do the work.

The true way to raise standards is not actually about homogenisation. It is to 'cut off the tail' of the quality curve. You have far more success if you simply stop amateur dabblers. Snuffing out the duffers makes overall standards shoot up. They are a far bigger threat to quality and safety than the majority of decent honest radiologists.

It is entirely possible to have quite a lot of variation in a technique and still sit atop the quality curve. This gets at the heart of this rule. Despite endless exhortations to do a radiological scan or procedure in one particular specific way, it is not always necessary to do it the same way. In fact, there are many advantages to not doing so. The caveat is that you must know what you are doing. It has to be a deliberate decision.

I'll give you an example. Standards documents state that you should do a CTC in two opposite positions—prone and supine. The problem is that old folk sometimes cannot lie comfortably on their front. And plump people squish all their colon with their body weight in that position. So after a bit of thinking, we decided to perform both scans with the older and/or plumper patient lying on first left and then right side. It works a treat. You get a better quality scan and the patient is more comfortable.

There are options just like this for every single procedure or scan that we radiologists do. There are ways to improve the quality of the procedure without compromising the patient experience. Or, more importantly, there are ways of improving the patient experience without compromising the quality of the procedure.

This is why experience and expertise are so, so important in the investigational arts. It is unfeasible to capture all the subtleties and nuances of expertise in a written protocol. Hands-on experience of doing the same thing thousands of times over many years to a wide variety of patients produces a unique professional.

The difference in this unique professional is that because they are doing the procedure on complete auto-pilot, they can afford the luxury of listening to the patient. They get additional medical history direct from the patient, often different to that stated on the request card. It allows them to individualise the procedure, the very antithesis of a 'sausage factory' approach. Patients should never feel like a piece of meat on a production line.

The most horrible mistakes can arise if the radiologist doesn't talk to the patient. The worst case scenario is where patients draw their last breath during a diagnostic procedure. I've been there. It is deeply upsetting and wrong on so many levels. So, preferably before you get started, talk to the patient and use your clinical reasoning. At the very least you'll avoid accidental forays into peri-mortem imaging. This topic is so important that you can read all about it in Rule #64.

Chapter 35
Rule #35 / / If You Have To Fail, Fail Safely

Struggling is learning. But only to the point that adrenaline turns brown. Recognize your boundaries and approach them cautiously, with the cavalry in the wings.

—

I should rephrase this Rule as '*When* you fail, fail safely' as it isn't a question of *if* but more *when*. Error, mistakes and failure are an inescapable part of life; radiology is no exception to this (see Rules #32 and #50). Sometimes it is 100% an accidental lapse or fumble. This happens to the best of us. Occasionally people 'get cute'; exhibiting risky behaviour to save time as they are phenomenally busy. Deliberate recklessness or a cavalier approach is very rare in my experience.

The vast majority of cases are not entirely the fault of the individual. It is often a combination of factors. It might be a high risk patient or a bit of kit that fails at a crucial moment (typically at 4am). In the NHS you can assume the physical environment isn't exactly conducive either. For NHS you can read any other underfunded healthcare environment.

If you take a scientific approach to error (and there are those who do just that) there are three broad categories of reasons for error. These are (1) the individual; (2) their working environment and (3) the organisation in which they work. These three pillars of Human Factors also form the holy triumvirate of error.

There is another model of error that gets everywhere. You cannot go to a talk about error in radiology without this image popping up. The model is a piece of cheese with holes in it. Termed the 'Swiss Cheese' model, it was dreamt up by James Reason in 2000. If I was to let my inner pedant speak, I'd call it the 'Emmental' model. This is simply because any self-respecting turophile knows that Vacherin, Raclette, Gruyere and the other 99% of Swiss cheeses are quite hole-free.

Anyway, no matter. Our hero Dr Reason saw slices of cheese as the defences against error. Each slice represents a different person, a safety process, a barrier of

P. McCoubrie, *The Rules of Radiology*, https://doi.org/10.1007/978-3-030-65229-6_35

some kind. It is an odd analogy, if you think about it. Cheese isn't normally used in defence. I suppose a particularly ripe Camembert left unwrapped in a warm room can deter all but the most determined of interlopers. But it'd be a strange world where hospitals mounted a cheese-based system of patient safety.

I digress. The key feature is that every slice of Emmental contains holes (technically called 'eyes', if you are interested). The holes represent vulnerabilities in the defence against error or 'latent conditions'. These represent natural flaws in any system, person or process. Normally these holes are offset from one another. With enough slices, there is usually a complete barrier to error. But just occasionally there are enough holes in several adjacent slices that line up and allow error to occur.

This model has advantages in that it embraces complexity. It defocuses on individuals and looks at all the factors that allowed the error to happen. This is crucial. It is easy and natural for the crooked finger of blame to point at individuals. This turns safety investigations into witch hunts. The outcome is the burning of the accused at the stake. Or, in the modern world, disciplinary action.

If you want people to learn when something has gone wrong, you don't look for witches to burn. You look at broad picture. You look at all the 'latent conditions' or holes in the cheese. And you try and fix them. Or add an extra layers of defence/cheese. You most certainly can over-react to latent conditions. If you add too many layers of safety, you become so rule-bound that your staff can barely get anything done, such are the sheer numbers of mandatory checks and balances.

The Emmental model doesn't always work. Sometimes things go wrong due to a single point of failure. The risk or latent condition is often unknown before the error happens. They aren't known fallibilities. There is no rhyme or reason to the errors. There is no root cause after analysis. You can't prevent them through any systematic improvement or learning endeavour. They just happen sporadically, irrespective of preparedness, skill, experience or vigilance (see Rule #32).

I'll give you an example: me, this morning. I arrived at work to discover my keys were missing. I retraced my steps and eventually found them 40 min later, still in the lock of my own front door. Lord alone knows what I was thinking. Well, I clearly wasn't thinking. It isn't incompetence at door locking. For several thousand consecutive days prior to this I have quite successfully locked my front door, deposited my keys in my pocket and cycled to work.

I should reassure you that despite this temporary aberration I'm not particularly hare-brained or other-worldly. I do know plenty of radiologists who are terminally disorganised. They seem to be surrounded by a minor sphere of chaos and leave a trail of disorganisation behind them. I even trained with someone who was so scatterbrained that it amounted an aberration of space–time. They were affected by an Uncertainty Principle as they were never in the same place as their phone *and* keys simultaneously.

Anyway, there is a attractive concept that bridges the complexity of error covering both simple glitches and multi-cause failures. This the notion of 'Just Culture'. When I first heard of it, I thought it was just a brand of plain yoghurt. Which, of course, it isn't. But if you've not come across it before, do have a closer look. It doesn't seek to blame the system for failures of individuals yet it doesn't blame the individual for system failures. It also doffs its hat to accountability. It differentiates a simple mistake by a conscientious professional from a preventable error made by a reckless incompetent.

This backdrop of cheese and not-a-yoghurt may sound like patient safety experts are dairy-obsessed. But I am told this is a happy coincidence. It does indicate that there are some clever types out there who take error in healthcare very seriously. Indeed they have been doing so for many decades. I must admit it annoys me when the media wail about the lack of attention paid to patient safety in modern healthcare. It just isn't true.

Focusing on patient safety through systematic prevention of error is actually relatively easy when you are dealing with low-risk and planned procedures. Through systematic improvements and training of individuals you can make safe procedures even safer. But it is more difficult to keep a close eye on error in high-risk and urgent procedures. Normally this involves a very poorly patient who needs urgently sorting out. Safety takes a back seat in such unplanned or emergency situations.

The traditional model of emergencies is that the heroic individual pulls out all the professional stops and saves the day. As we will see in Rule #82, the secret to success is very much the opposite. We should not rely on individuals in regularly performing earth-shattering acts. Firstly it is isn't reliable, secondly it isn't sustainable and, thirdly you are better with a team around you. There are many lessons from other safety–critical industries such as aviation that indicate that the higher the risk, the more urgent the scenario, the more we should actually rely on a protocol.

Protocols work well in regular safety–critical tasks. Our radiology department has a handful for the regular stuff, like communicating unexpected serious findings. Which can go badly wrong if you don't do everything by the book. But flying an aircraft is not the same as healthcare and the parallels between the two only go so far. Medicine is endlessly more complex, more nuanced, more varied than the airline industry. You cannot write protocols for all scenarios. One individual will be au fait with thousands of scenarios but each one will be subtly different and need a different tack. And no individual will be a slick expert in all the scenarios they encounter in a single working day. You would hope that, given time, it all gets rather routine and mundane as you master increasing parts of your working life.

After over 20 years in radiology I can safely say that mastery is a journey not a destination. I still struggle every day. This is because I encounter something new and unknown, or something vague and ill-defined or something that I once knew but have forgotten. It is for this reason that I can safely say, without sanctimony, that I am learning every day of my professional life. The more I struggle to master something, the more I learn. This old dog still learns lots of new tricks.

This is where this Rule kicks in. Trying to master something has its hazards. Because you are used to daily struggles, it is a fine line between grappling with a gritty problem and finding yourself out of your depth. Part of being a good radiologist is recognising these boundaries. Some call it situational awareness, some call it a gut instinct, some call it a Sixth Sense. Whatever you call it, don't ignore these cognitive alarm bells. Call for help, call for back up, ask for another opinion before things go wrong rather than after. Better to call them and not need them rather than call them too late.

Chapter 36
Rule #36 / / Take Clinical Details With A Pinch Of Salt

We were all junior doctors; we know why they write the clinical details that they do. We understand that clinical examination is fickle—the words 'shifting dullness' are 100% negatively predictive for ascites on ultrasound. We understand the pressures—'?SDH' on a CT Head card merely means the boss's ward round is looming. See Rule #37.

—

Doctors are, on the whole, a fairly honest bunch. Surveys show that we are one of the most trusted professions. This is no accident. All doctors have high moral standards drummed into them from Day One of medical school. We buy into this whole-heartedly: medical practice is close to a religion of morality. If asked to produce a self-portrait, most doctors would paint themselves as lily-white water-walkers who have their hand directly guided by the Almighty.

Anyone deviating from this sainted narrative of professional practice is ostracised. A proven lapse in moral standards sees that doctor ruthlessly run out of town. 'Bringing the profession into disrepute' is a frequent charge when doctors are struck off. Honesty, openness and trustworthiness are at the heart of this. Read the UK's General Medical Council publications and these buzzwords spring from every paragraph.

But the concept of absolute honesty is a flimsy house of cards. It doesn't bear close inspection. If I said to you that all doctors lie, you might be raise an eyebrow or two. If I added that I was lied to all day, every day, you might stroke your chin with intrigue. If I turned to you, dear reader, and accused even you of lying on a regular basis, you might wrinkle your nose in annoyance. But don't blame me. As appalling as this might seem, it is true.

Doctors can indeed be just as dishonest as, say, Tory Prime Ministers. Or U.S. Presidents. I'm not singling out doctors or politicians. Everyone lies to a certain degree, even those with the highest moral standards. As Groucho Marx observed,

"There is one way to find out if a man is honest—ask him. If he says 'yes', then he is a crook".

My problem is the self-righteousness. I came across this rather angry quote the other day, "When someone lies to you, it is because they don't respect you enough to be honest and they think you are too stupid to know the difference". I get it, I really do. No one likes finding out they've been lied to. But as virtually no-one is 100% scrupulously honest, it is hypocritical posturing.

There are those who have pushed the idea of uncompromising honesty. Immanuel Kant suggested this in a 1798 essay 'On a Supposed Right to Tell Lies from Benevolent Motives'. Several others have proposed something similar, the latest iteration being 'Radical Honesty'. They remain refreshing and interesting but most people find this moral code actually very difficult to live. After all, social graces and politeness are largely ritualistic lies.

Without lies, marriages would crumble, workers would be fired, egos would be shattered, governments would collapse. You'd never be able to say, 'Yes, let's definitely get together soon'. Men (and women) would have to be honest about their less socially acceptable physiological urges. And parenting of small children would be just about impossible.

The proof that everyone lies is not just anecdotes and conjecture. There are a wealth of psychological experiments, neatly summarized by Prof Dan Ariely in his very approachable book *The (Honest) Truth about Dishonesty*. I do recommend it as a fascinating read but there are a few interesting generalizations that he covers:

- First, minor dishonesty is ubiquitous, perhaps exemplified by white lies, "No, your bum doesn't look big in that".
- Second, most people feel fine with minor dishonesty; people cheat up to a level where they start to feel bad.
- Third, cheating is contagious. If others are cheating, you are more likely to cheat yourself. If you've already cheated, you are likely to cheat again.
- Fourth, many other factors increase the likelihood of dishonesty. For example, if you work somewhere where there is a culture of dishonesty, you are far more likely to be dishonest yourself.
- Fifth, major dishonesty is rare but is generally a slippery slope story. It starts with an initial act of dishonesty that, in certain circumstances, leads into a spiral of lies and deceit. You start off as a rational human and end up behaving like a borderline psychopath. But crucially, the individual rationalises this and sees no problem.

If absolute honesty is akin to cruelty but major dishonesty is psychopathic, what are we to do? As Oscar Wilde put it, "Morality is like art, you have to draw a line somewhere". Most of us would err towards truthfulness. After all 'not bearing false witness' is part of the Ten Commandments of Judeo-Christian tradition. Is it ever acceptable for a doctor to deliberately lie? Where is the line for radiologists?

I tend towards the scrupulously honest end of the spectrum. There is a simple reason for this. You never know when the thought police will come knocking. If (or rather *when*) I suffer a fall from grace, I want no skeletons in the cupboard.

If someone goes muckraking, they'll find nothing. It is self-protection. It has the added benefit of sleeping better at night.

I will admit that I have been occasionally less than truthful in my radiological practice. But I can put my hand on my heart and say it has never been for gain or self-advancement. I'll give you an example of a dilemma I've faced a number of times.

The scene—an ultrasound room, patient lies supine, I'm on the probe end of things, chatting away to the patient. Suddenly I find a cancer. I know with 99% certainty that it is cancer. The chat dries up, my demeanour changes (I am rubbish at a poker face). Spotting my concern, the patient asks, "What is wrong?". I am non-committal, explaining that, "we will have to do more tests" and other evasive statements.

Why do I do this? Well, in 1% of patients, it won't be cancer. It'll be one the many many conditions that mimic cancer. A sheep in wolf's clothing, as it were. It is one of the major reasons why radiologists pussyfoot over diagnoses. I've been there, utterly convinced it is cancer but remembering the times that I was wrong. Traditionally this turns out to be TB, sarcoid or HIV (but never lupus).

But the fear of being wrong isn't the main reason I dip my toes into the waters of dishonesty. It is for a good reason—the ultrasound couch is no place for breaking bad news. Once a patient hears the word 'cancer', they hear nothing else. I accidentally went there once and the patient's subsequent distress is seared into my memory.

Radiologists can give a useful 'shot across the bows', hinting to the patient that all is not well, which can be very useful when bad news is confirmed later. Of course this is done not for reasons of medical paternalism. It is actually part of compassionate care. A slightly gloomy but non-specific message to the patient about their scan allows bad news to be broken appropriately, done in discrete stages.

There you go. I have bared my soul. I am no saint. For this reason I don't expect other doctors to be irreproachably pure. I imagine that most radiologists are in exactly the same position. We understand the pressures of the clinical work-place. Specifically, we know that there are unwritten rules of radiology requesting. Clinicians always ask for scans in a particular way. This method of asking is the same the world over; an absolute invariant between clinician and radiology services. It isn't how you ask, it is the clinical details you write on the request form.

The overall goal is get the scan done as soon as possible with the minimum of fuss. The first step is to ensure that your request is accepted. To do this you must write sufficient details indicating the patient is unwell enough to warrant a scan. The second step is to ensure the scan is prioritised over others. The medical details must therefore hint at a disease process that needs rapid assessment. The third step is that you must do all this without being dishonest and thus beyond reproach.

Obviously if the patient is unwell then no games or gambits are necessary. The facts are stated plainly, radiologist snaps to it and the patient gets a urgent scan. The difficulties arise when the patient is not unwell. At this point the clinician has decisions to make. Are they honest and risk the scan either being bounced or demoted to a low priority? Or do they fib a little to get the scan accepted and / or done promptly?

Most radiologists deploy a bullshit filter when they read radiology requests. They know the clinical details are a version of the truth. When faced with a daily torrent of half-truths on radiology requests, it is very easy to become distraught. Nihilistic, even. However, you mustn't take it personally. I've seen many radiologists broken on this particular hill.

A radiologist must therefore take all requests with a pinch of salt. By doing this, you protect yourself from being ground down by the daily torrent of bent truths. Furthermore, you become adept at spotting who is genuinely ill and actually needs a scan, as opposed to the majority who aren't and can safely wait.

Chapter 37
Rule #37 / / Don't Crap On Juniors

You can judge a doctor by how they treat those lower on the medical ladder. Those on the lower rungs need a hand up. A radiologist can provide help and education. Education, however, can be delivered pretty assertively. Especially at 3 am. See Rules #2, #3, #9 and #36.

—

One of the downsides of a medical career is the sheer length of the training. I spent 15 years as a student and junior doctor. Before you reach for a violin I should say that I had an absolute blast. It is one of the upsides of being a 'work hard; play hard' sort of fella. But it meant sacrifices galore. By the age of 50 most doctors have already put in the same hours that others do during their whole working life. Which might explain why I feel so damned knackered.

Most of the bosses I had were supportive and pretty egalitarian. I felt valued despite my junior status and varying degrees of incompetence. Now that I am a boss myself, I try to pay this forward by being kind to those lower down the career ladder. They need a hand up. I also try to be equally kind and supportive to all, irrespective of their status or profession.

It isn't easy. When you are busy, social niceties go out of the window. If you have no time and lots to do, you don't want to faff around. You want to speak to the organ grinder, not the monkey. But you should be absolutely civil about this. When I was the medical equivalent of a small dancing simian in a fez, I didn't mind others bypassing me to go straight to the boss provided they were polite.

Being blanked or treated as invisible was quite common. The more junior you were, the more invisible you were. But it wasn't a big problem. I understood that not everyone is gregarious and socially confident. I understood that not everyone thinks of others before themself. I understood that people can have a lot on their mind, sometimes too much to consider social graces.

Not that we didn't lap it up when we were treated nicely by someone higher up the food chain. You were chuffed to bits if they even bothered to ask your name

P. McCoubrie, *The Rules of Radiology*, https://doi.org/10.1007/978-3-030-65229-6_37

rather than just calling you 'Boy' or 'Oi, you there'. Just occasionally they took an interest, went out of their way to be kind and it made your day. I remember those transient snippets, those fleeting pleasantries. They made all the privations of the junior doctor years a little more bearable.

I will admit that by the time I reached my last years of training I had had enough of being a junior doctor. Some of my colleagues were filled with terror at the prospect of being a consultant whereas I couldn't wait. Although technically a junior doctor, I was in my early 30 s and had more letters after my name than in it. I was sick of kowtowing to people purely based on their seniority.

Of course I didn't mind doffing my cap and tugging a forelock to those that deserved respect. They might not have been very nice people but they were undeniably good at what they did. I would positively prostrate myself if they were both a decent sort and highly talented. But as the years rolled on, I had increasing difficulty in showing faux respect for senior doctors that didn't deserve it, either because they weren't actually very good or they were uncivil. Often both.

I didn't mind the ones that were a bit duff but perfectly pleasant. We can't all be Nobel Prize winners. Some of them might have been hotshots when they were younger but were now distinctly lukewarm. They had rested on their laurels for so long that the leaves had positively fossilised. But most were honest and friendly so you could still learn a trick or two from them.

There is a natural rhythm to a medical career, a sine wave of potency, an ebb and flow of competence. There comes a stage in one's professional life where you are no longer in ascendency. Most accept this inevitable gentle decline gracefully, moving from mid-career pomp to late-career decorum. Radiologists are less prone to this than the craft specialities. Sixty-five year old radiologists are usually still pretty damn handy but a surgeon of the same vintage has lost much of their physical prowess.

I trained under several older radiologists who had difficulty coping with this. Blind to their waning powers, they kidded themselves that they knew everything still. And they went down raging, raging against the dying of the light. If they couldn't be top dog anymore, no one else could be. They expressed their dissatisfaction by taking pot-shots at those junior to them. Their vitriol was particularly reserved for those that threatened to shatter the illusion of their competence by doing ridiculous things like, I dunno, questioning things, exhibiting competence and being assertive.

There was another type that got up my nose. This was the 'Mr Darcy'. Not so much the character from *Bridget Jones* but the original from Austen's *Pride and Prejudice*. This mildly disagreeable type is proud and arrogant. Their feeling of superiority leads to haughty or condescending sarcasm. They are, of course, largely civil but they cannot conceal their abhorrence of having to deal with lesser individuals.

I have no problem with sarcasm. None whatsoever: I'm a Brit, after all. Light-hearted banter, sarcasm, irony and ridicule are natural to British folk as much as breathing and eating. And this is important. We Brits strongly believe that nothing is sacrosanct. If it exists, we take the mickey out of it. But there is a unwritten rule—always aim it upwards.

We take the piss out of those higher up the ladder to puncture their pomposity, to arraign their arrogance. It is a great leveller of hierarchies. But it is very unBritish to be sarcastic towards those junior to yourself. In fact, it is usually the hallmark of a bully. Or a grasping narcissist, only interested in themselves, their power and their wealth. So those who crap on juniors should be judged negatively. I don't often advocate a negative stance but feel on pretty safe ground here.

Perhaps it doesn't need saying but it is very poor form to use 'hard' sarcasm. Sarcasm that is intended to denigrate, undermine or deliberately offend has no role in the workplace. This is why sarcasm should be used cautiously, sparingly and softly. Try to use it with people who you know can take a ribbing. You'll get fewer formal complaints that way. When Oscar Wilde wrote, 'Sarcasm is the lowest form of wit but the highest form of intelligence', he understood the dilemma inherent using it.

I have a problem with hierarchies in medicine. Given that we are social creatures, you cannot eliminate hierarchies entirely. There will always be a pecking order. I remember being bottom of the heap. The heap is composed entirely of people who remember exactly what it was like when they were at the bottom, but who have put on a lot of weight as they've clambered upwards.

There is a very good reason to deliberately erode hierarchies. The concept of 'hierarchy gradients' was first used in aviation safety. A flat gradient indicates equality in a team; a steep gradient indicates a strong divide between the haves and have nots. Psychologists quickly recognised that strong cockpit hierarchies were a factor in many plane crashes. One of the biggest problems was that the other crew couldn't question a captain's dodgy decisions.

The parallels in medicine and radiology are huge. Ensuring that all members of the healthcare team have a voice is the main reason to flatten hierarchies whenever possible. Put simply, flat hierarchies save lives.

So. We don't punch down, we are kind and supportive to all, we reduce hierarchies through humour. Should be straightforward, shouldn't it? But, as is often the case, fine words butter no parsnips. Radiologists don't do this often enough. Rightly or wrongly, radiologists are seen as grumpy and unhelpful. I hope that full-on abuse of junior doctors is rare but certainly we often are directly responsible for decreasing their quality of life. So how does a radiologist do this whilst remaining both sane and productive?

I find that folk just want it straight. If you are doing the scan, they want to know when. If not, they want to know why not? I try to turn this negative into a positive. A simple polite explanation is often all that is required but it could be a teaching opportunity or a chance for some pertinent feedback if they've got something wrong.

Although feedback is a dark and difficult art, radiologists should avoid negative judgements of the requesting clinician. Don't say, "You blithering idiot, do you realise it is 4 am?"; say, "It isn't indicated now. We'll do the scan at 8 am". Don't say, "This is a pile of crap, are you even medically qualified?"; say, "Sounds a difficult case. Maybe your consultant could call me when they've seen the patient?".

The most difficult encounter is the aggressive clinician. But you'll have to read onto Rule #38 to find out about that.

Chapter 38
Rule #38 / / Aggressive Clinicians Need Your Help

If a doctor gets rude and shouty, they are usually (i) out of their depth, (ii) unsupported and (iii) worried about their patient. See past the emotion and try to help. Persistent offenders need showing the door and reminding, "My scanner, not your scanner". See Rule #3.

—

I've never been physically assaulted. Well, not since I was nineteen. But that was my brother and we were both drunk, so it doesn't count. Since then I've barely even been lightly jostled. Perhaps it is because most would-be aggressors think twice about tackling 100 kg of Yorkshire Beef. My physical bulk notwithstanding, I suspect many radiologists are in the same boat. For that we are can consider ourselves rather fortunate.

Assaults on healthcare staff are virtually always by a patient. Makes sense, really. Any doctor who gets a bit punchy would be defrocked faster than you can say 'antidisestablishmentarianism'. Physical assaults on staff by patients make me sick to my stomach. Patients may be delirious or have dementia but assaults by cognitively intact patients are inexcusable.

Verbal assaults are another thing. Sadly these are not infrequent in the hospital world. We radiologists are often on the receiving end of these. Overt verbal aggression is rare. I am struggling to think of the last time someone shouted at me in the workplace. Gratuitous and deliberately hurtful insults are also pretty damn uncommon. But low-grade unpleasantness is common, even in a hospital like mine which prides itself on be a relatively civil place to work.

I was chatting with a clinical colleague the other day when I ventured that the most difficult part of being a radiologist was dealing with an aggressive and rude clinician. They pshawed at this, countering they'd been on the receiving end from radiologists far more often than they'd ever dished it out.

As a general rule, most individuals think that they are on the sharp end more often than others. The reasons for this are fairly simple. We are all prone to

P. McCoubrie, *The Rules of Radiology*, https://doi.org/10.1007/978-3-030-65229-6_38

cognitive bias. There is a specific form of recall bias where we disproportionately remember the worst aspects of any occasion. This means that any negativity can taint an otherwise positive episode. This is true whether this is chatting to a radiologist, having a colonoscopy or enduring a visit from the mother-in-law.

The other cognitive bias centres around egocentricity. Now not every hospital doctor is excessively conceited. There are varying degrees. I've worked with solipsists; those whose world-view is utterly self-centred. They barely register other humans. Proper conversation is lacking as they don't listen. They look at others like they don't really exist. You may be thinking that I am referring to surgeons but I couldn't possibly comment.

The ego-driven individual believes they are blessed with excellent social skills. This might be true but most of us are blind to our own foibles. Again, the Kruger-Dunning effect delivers a beautiful irony here. Those with the social skills of a rutting rhino over-rate their abilities whilst those that are smoother than a buttered fox are secretly wracked with self-doubt.

Funnily enough egotists give radiologists little trouble. We barely register on their radar; we are just another talking ghost to them. They only give us trouble when they find themselves reliant on a radiology opinion. And then radiologists experience outbursts of snooty arrogance and belittling behaviour as their ego seeks to exert itself. Radiologists have been there, seen that, bought the t-shirt, worn it out, now use it as a duster. We brush off their nonsense like pie crumbs from a silk tie.

I've reflected on aggressiveness amongst clinicians. It can happen when a consultation with a clinician goes south. As we saw in Rule #30, this may or may not be your fault. Avoid this at all costs. Everyone loses if radiologists argue with a clinician. Especially the patient.

The most common form of aggression is microaggression. These are usually thoughtless and minor acts: a snide comment here, a passive-aggressive snip there, and everywhere low-grade hostility. Most of us become fairly immune to these demeaning mini-insults. But even a paper cut can still be annoying. Death by 1000 paper cuts is not just an abstract concept; your soul leaches out via the epidermis.

It is very different to assertiveness or grumpiness. The micro-aggressor has ignored the memo about being kind and polite. They typically belong to a socially dominant group. There is often a swaggering machismo to their medical practice. It seems like everything is a giant game and that they somehow have to win. Their mothers would not be proud of them.

This behaviour is affected by institutional norms. It is more commonly seen in large university teaching hospitals and rarer in smaller district general hospitals. Don't mislabel this as a 'sick building' syndrome; the bricks and mortar are blameless. It is also speciality and department specific. Individual groups or whole departments often been habitually rude for years without any challenge. Not only are they rude to everyone else but usually horrifically rude to each other. It is the tone laid down by senior clinicians and managers who unwittingly allow a toxic culture to be perpetuated.

There is no easy answer to microaggresion amidst a toxic culture. I've seen people drawn into it, previously decent people who start working in such an environment who gradually become toxic themselves. The first step is insight. It is difficult to be objective about your immediate environment but certainly possible. Once you have gained insight then higher professional standards are easier. Clear social boundaries are emancipatory. You must rise above it all. Do not stoop to their level; do not offer to wrestle with a pig (see Rule #30).

The most important type of aggressive clinician is one whose worry and frustration manifests as anger. I get this. It is difficult to remain rational when a patient is dying right in front of you, you don't know why and no one seems able or willing to help. To literally scream with full-throated passion is quite understandable.

This consultation is one of the most difficult. Trying to help someone that is rude and aggressive is a great test of professionalism. The natural reaction is to retaliate, to fight fire with fire. Again, don't. You must remain calm (see Rule #3).

This aggression can be difficult to distinguish from straightforward unpleasantness. It could just be a normal clinician having a bit of a moment. Clinicians that are a 'bit of a character' (i.e. a bullying dick) can also be worried about a patient. Hence anyone that is being an objectionable arse could actually need your help.

I see this happening predominantly in the middle of the night. One of our nightshift registrars recently told me a story of an aggressive and rude clinician making unreasonable demands at 5am. But then my clinical colleagues told me of an equally unhelpful and obstructive night-shift registrar. It is almost like two different scenarios, such are the disparities.

It doesn't need a PhD in psychology to work out what went wrong. If the young clinician or radiologist is dog-tired, they are vulnerable. More so if working without direct supervision. Add in varying degrees of inexperience, being busy as hell, a lengthening queue of sick patients and it is enough to almost break anyone. The straw on the camel's back is another doctor who is less than civil at 5 am. Surprised it doesn't happen more often, actually.

So what does a radiologist do with an aggressive clinician? The first step is de-escalation. It is mainly verbal but there are non-verbal elements too. Invite them to sit but allow personal space. Adopt an open and relaxed posture. Force a passable smile.

I'll summarise a few verbal pointers:

(1)   *Listen.* Allow them to vent. Only allow fifteen seconds though (see Rule #48).
(2)   *Acknowledge.* Legitimise the emotion but don't excuse the behavior.
(3)   *Agree.* Acknowledge the truth in their tirade. It snuffs out anger.
(4)   *Apologise.* Even if you've done nothing wrong, find something. It's hard to be angry at an apologist.
(5)   *Clarify.* Always worth being absolutely sure before judging.
(6)   *Choices.* Don't mandate the outcome. Suggest options.

They don't have to be any particular order, so long as the listening bit is toward the beginning and it ends in choices. I frequently diffuse the tension with a combination of 2–4 as an opening gambit such as, "Sorry to keep you waiting, have a seat; you look busy, is it hell out there?".

Most of the time this will work as there are very few persistently unpleasant clinicians out there. Just decent ones having a bit of a low moment. We all say or do things that we regret. Lord knows I've sinned this way but I have repented and tried to be a better human being. However, repeated aggressiveness and rudeness in the workplace is inexcusable whatever their grade, speciality, time of day, circumstance or clinical urgency. This is true for all hospital staff.

Every time a specific clinician is anti-social, I am making a mental withdrawal from their account in my Bank of Goodwill (see Rule #10). They can make a deposit any time by being pleasant. However, my overdraft limit is low. Those who try to make unauthorised withdrawals get pulled up. I tell them politely but firmly that their behaviour is unacceptable, reminding them it is 'my scanner, not yours' (or words to that effect).

Chapter 39
Rule #39 / / Know Loads

The job of the radiologist is to explain every pixel. Not just hazard a guess, but to know categorically. If you can't explain something, you aren't as good as you thought you were. See Rule #4.

—

Professor Paul Goddard is never short of opinions. Now retired, PG was a infamous radiologist at the Bristol Royal Infirmary. I spent many hours at his knee as a registrar, largely as the hospital couldn't afford chairs. I was fond of his irascible contrarian nature. He often regaled us with his firmly held beliefs, often encapsulated into aphorisms. He had no fear of poking fun at authority and tweaking the nose of orthodox thinking. His passion for questioning the status quo resonated with me. In a bygone age we would have both been strung up as blasphemous heretics.

One of his maxims has stuck with me. He postulated that, "Radiologists should be able to explain absolutely everything on the image". On first inspection this looks innocuous enough. He is merely urging radiologists to have deep understanding of the task in hand. The more you can explain, the better a radiologist you are. The corollary is that if you cannot do this then you aren't as clever as you thought you were.

There is another way of looking at this statement. If it is true then it implies that everything on the image can be explained; everything on the image has an explicable reason for being there. This is, in essence, the philosophical concept of objectivism. This view of social reality asserts that there are absolute truths. That is to say that at the heart of every matter lies a kernel of pure and incontrovertible knowledge.

It is a reassuring point of view; the ontological equivalent of warm maternal hug. It is a message of hope. Everything has an explanation and one of the goals of the human race is finding answers. It also indicates that if something is not currently known, it is only a matter of time before we can explain it. It is the

P. McCoubrie, *The Rules of Radiology*, https://doi.org/10.1007/978-3-030-65229-6_39

imperative behind scientific endeavour. It ensures that empirical science is central to the future of humanity.

The other end of this thought spectrum is constructivism. Unlike the certainty of objectivism, this holds that all is subjective. All knowledge about the world is highly individualised. There is no such thing as an ultimate truth as our perceptions and understanding of it colours it. Our understanding is a construct; it is constructed from experience. Each construct is different as it is influenced by our unique personal circumstances.

Bertrand Russell illustrates this in his classic *The Problems of Philosophy* with a lengthy exposition about, of all things, a table and Bismark, the first Chancellor of the German Empire. The table is a physical object which can be directly detected by our senses but is slightly different to each person that views or touches it, depending on the lighting, view point and so on. Bismark definitely existed but can only be understood indirectly through the explanation of others. This concept of direct and indirect 'knowing' is rather critical.

You see radiologists only know disease from visual data. Our understanding of disease is uni-sensory and therefore largely indirect. Other doctors have the advantage of four additional senses to call upon. Although as Richard Gordon's archetypal surgeon Sir Lancelot Spratt memorably instructed his students in *Doctor in the House*, 'Eyes first and most, hands next and least and tongue not at all'. Interestingly he omits any mention of listening. Which proves that surgeons haven't changed much in the last seventy years.

Constructivism disconcerts doctors. We generally believe that, for example, unobserved trees fall noisily. If someone told us of the notion that reality is a social invention then we would suspect them of mental illness. Should Laurence Fishburne suddenly manifest as Morpheus and proffer a choice of two pills, we'd probably all take the blue one.

It isn't surprising. Our medical training makes us this way. We are fed a steady diet of hard facts. We steadily ingest empirical data throughout our career. We are explicitly taught to think in a convergent fashion to clinch a single diagnosis (and squeal with delight when we are able to do so). The fact that single, pure diagnoses are rare and that real life is more like Donald Schön's 'swampy lowlands, where situations are confusing messes incapable of technical solution'.

Chuck a radiologist into a foreign field of study, such as the social sciences, and it feels very alien. I did just this when I studied for a Masters in Medical Education. The thinking here is divergent. It aims to generate multiple possible answers in an attempt to find one that works. The data is largely qualitative not quantitative. Conclusions require reasoning rather than statistical analysis. It was one of the mentally taxing but most serendipitous things I've ever done.

Once you've been a doctor for decades you forget how other non-doctors think. You become blind that there are other ways of thinking. The worst is that you disparage others who don't think like you. Studying a humanity opened my eyes as to how the other half of the world is trained to think. Moreover, it irreversibly changed how I saw the world. It was truly transformative.

These revelations, as it turns out, are far from original. CP Snow's *Two Cultures* in 1959 drew attention to the gaping chasm between those from a scientific background and those from a humanities or arts background. Far more impressive to me is the late and great Stephen Jay Gould. His erudition and unique fusion of science, the arts and history make him the best essayist bar none. His collections of essays are some of the most exciting books on the planet. *The Hedgehog, the Fox and the Magister's Pox* from 2003 shows the benefits that scientists can gain from the humanities and vice versa.

I'm not advocating that radiologists need to formally study the arts and humanities. That isn't the point. What I am arguing is that radiologists benefit from knowledge of different models of thinking. Having mental flexibility is a real advantage in tackling real-life problems. Explaining every pixel on an image needs more than just a deep knowledge of facts. But factual knowledge is the *sine qua non* of an expert radiologist.

An in-depth knowledge of the body, disease and it's radiological appearances is absolutely critical. It is why, bizarrely, most radiology books have more words than pictures. Radiology isn't just pattern recognition. Well, some of it is. But a small percentage. It is a unique visual expertise backed up by vast knowledge.

You need knowledge as you simply cannot see what you do not understand. If you have never heard of something, you cannot recognise it. You brain simply doesn't register it; the visual data is there but doesn't enter your consciousness as it is filtered out. The visual cortices make up some thirty percent of the brain, far more than hearing or touch. But eighty percent of the visual cortical connections are with other parts of the brain. Visual processing is heavily influenced by memories.

This quirk of visual processing has been called the 'Rumpelstiltskin phenomenon', after the fairy tale where a miller's daughter learns the name of the imp that has tormented her and thereby gains power over him. The notion is that once you know the name of something and you understand it, you have power over it. This is true in radiology. You cannot spot conditions that you've never heard of.

A good radiologist needs book-based medical knowledge. Lots of it. It is why post-graduate training is so long and arduous. The radiologist needs to know the body from top to bottom, back to front, inside out—a radiologist can never know too much anatomy (see Rule #44). You need to know the common everyday stuff but you need to be aware of the small print stuff too (see Rule #54).

The best radiologists seem to know everything. Of course they don't but the best ones are walking medical encyclopedias. The last person judged to know everything was the polymath (and doctor) Thomas Young. He died in 1823 aged 56 after having usurped Newton with his wave theory of light, coined Young's modulus and as if that wasn't enough, found time to translate the Rosetta Stone amongst his many achievements.

Facts alone don't describe everything. They can take you only so far. The convergent-thinking, objectivist, empiricist is lost at the radiological coal face. In real life, little is certain. Multiple disease processes are common and establishing a firm single diagnosis is rather rare. Therefore a radiologist needs to be able to flip into a more divergent mode of thinking, generating possible explanations and using reason to come to a most likely diagnosis.

The best radiologists already do this. But it isn't explicit. If you ask them how they generate their diagnoses, most wouldn't be able to explain it. They just do it instinctively. They use their vast knowledge flexibly and vary their diagnostic thinking to match the task in hand. And then they communicate this slickly. Which is where Thomas Young would have made a poor radiologist. He may have been the living embodiment of the Renaissance but was famously unable to communicate his notions to lesser mortals.

And this, dear reader, is why being a good radiologist is so bloody hard.

Chapter 40
Rule #40 // Never Offer To Eat Your Pants

You might be so totally convinced in your diagnostic accuracy that you offer to do something silly if you are wrong. Sure as eggs are eggs, you will be tasting cloth sooner than you think.

———

I had been a consultant for a year when I offered to eat my underpants. I should probably point out that it isn't something I routinely offer. And, hitherto, I'd never ingested clothing of any sort. I remember the occasion very clearly, as if it has been seared into my hippocampus. As Plutarch wrote, "those who receive with the most pains and difficulty, remember best; every new thing they learn being, as it were, burnt and branded on their minds."

The occasion when this arose concerned discussion of a scan of an elderly chap who was known to have prostate cancer. For some reason he'd had a CT of the head which showed a mass in the outer membranes of the brain (the meninges). It was exerting some pressure on the underlying brain. I thought it was entirely typical for a meningioma, a type of benign brain tumour.

A reasonable assumption, you might have thought. Meningiomas are the most common meningeal tumour in this age group. They are common incidental findings but can cause pressure symptoms. My mistake wasn't assuming it was a meningioma. My mistake was swearing blind that it was a meningioma. I was so convinced that I haughtily refuted any other diagnosis. I snorted derisively at the notion of it being a metastasis from his prostate cancer.

At that time I had never heard of prostate cancer spreading to the meninges. I knew some tumours could do so but I had not heard of prostate cancer doing this. My error was assuming that if I had not heard of it then it couldn't be so. In fact, such was my self-confidence that when I presented the radiological findings at an x-ray meeting that I claimed that I would consume my underwear if it turned out to be a prostate metastasis. Of course, I learned afterwards that prostate cancer can spread to the meninges. It is extremely rare but well described.

157
P. McCoubrie, *The Rules of Radiology*, https://doi.org/10.1007/978-3-030-65229-6_40

Just two weeks later one of the clinicians turned up to the self-same clinico-ra-diological meeting with a smirk on his face. He told me that the patient went for surgery and the resected mass was a prostate metastasis and, unless he was mis-taken, that I had sworn blind that this couldn't be so and that I should start devour-ing my undies.

At this stage I knew I had fallen off my pedestal. When anyone starts in post they are placed on a metaphorical pedestal. They are the bright new hope. Fresh blood in a radiology department is a treasured thing. It is something to be cele-brated. Mainly as a colleague without overt cynicism is rather novel. We marvel at their brightness of their eyes and bushiness of their tails.

The intrinsic problems with being on a pedestal are (i) the pressure of expec-tation and (ii) sadly, there is only one way off it. Eventually, despite your best efforts, you will take a nose dive. Everyone will slip, stumble or slither eventually. Error is ever-present in radiology and no radiologist is immune (see Rule #50). I had been warned about this. Now the advice I give is, "When you fall from grace, fall gracefully".

And this is the point of this Rule. These Rules are a letter to my younger self. I'm telling other people about my mistakes so that they don't have to make them. So if you are a young radiologist, take these hints and tips from an older radi-ologist. If you are an older radiologist, use The Rules to help your younger col-leagues. If you aren't a radiologist, be kind to them as some won't have read The Rules.

Radiology departments can be very small places, especially when you make a diagnostic boo-boo. Colleagues flock because they want to learn from it: mistakes are there to be learnt from (see Rule #51). They also are watching for what hap-pens next. It isn't curiosity in the comeuppance of a colleague. Well, maybe a bit. But it is mainly as you learn a lot about the new kid from how they behave after they've fluffed up.

After the underpant incident I was mortified. I ate huge portions of humble pie. I reeled my neck right in. But not everyone does the same. Some lash out and blame others. Some double down and argue that others must be wrong. The more that they wriggle and squirm, the worse a radiologist they are. The enlightened radiologist says only one thing when they are told of a mistake: "Thank you." It is the only correct response.

On this occasion the clinicians were very gentle about this. They realised it was the hubris of the young and over-confident. My radiology colleagues were kind about my bumblings. This was a great balm to a young consultant who was finding his feet. I have subsequently tried to pay this forward by being similarly under-standing to my younger colleagues when they, in turn, plunge from their plinths.

The last thing you want after a semi-public humiliation is your colleagues being unpleasant about it. I once trained in a fairly hostile department. It was a veritable viper's nest where certain radiologists behaved quite malignantly. Mistakes were seized upon and used as chess pieces in power battles. The clin-ical director complained about being unable to turn around in narrow corridors due to the number of knives in their back. Funnily enough they had difficulty with recruitment and retention.

Most radiology departments are very supportive of those who've made a mistake. It is dealt with sensitively. The individual is supported as they explore what happened and what can be learnt. An open and honest ethos allows a positive to arise from a negative. This is enlightened behaviour.

A gentle teasing is to be expected; welcome, even. The reaction should match the degree of error. When it is a serious event and someone comes to harm, then you are tactful and supportive to your colleague. Be cautious with your light ribbing, probably not the time or place. If it is a minor transgression where no one came to harm, then expect your colleagues to queue up to take the piss. Then never drop it, ever.

Humour is a good way of keeping it light. I'm not sure I could have coped so easily if a colleague had over-analysed it and taken me aside for a Serious Chat. I would have really started doubting my own abilities. Many radiologists don't need help in this. They often abreact on discovering they've made an error. It's the perfectionist streak that most medics have.

A dip in confidence in one's abilities is normal reaction after making an error. When you've been professionally knocked down it takes a while to get back up. But get back up you must and preferably stronger than before, having learnt. Allowing error to wound you, to puncture your bubble of self-belief is a big mistake. A radiologist who loses their bottle is on a slippery slope into uselessness. You simply must retain trust your own judgement.

Obviously, there is a balance to be found. You don't want to be the radiologist that is 'often wrong but never in doubt'. Bluffers are bloody liabilities. Nobody wants a pig-headed colleague who makes a vague guess and then refuses to change their opinion despite mounting evidence to the contrary. They are lying to themself and others. And a dishonest radiologist is a dangerous radiologist.

On the other end of the spectrum is the radiologist who has totally lost faith in their judgement. I've worked with some spectacularly under-confident radiologists. The fear of being wrong robs them of the joy of being right. They sit on the fence so often that their backside is perpetually peppered with splinters. They hedge, they are vague, they are over-inclusive and non-committal. Their reports are, in a word, crap. They are the antithesis of clinically useful.

Under-confident radiologists are far more common that over-confident ones. I don't think it is a gender thing or anything to do with one's cultural heritage. If that were true, it'd be the other way around as UK radiology is currently male-heavy. But it isn't what radiologists want to be. They want to be sensible, measured and give a sound opinion. We are trained to solve problems and give a definitive answer.

I have two theories about why so many radiologists are under-confident and churn out wishy-washy reports. It isn't because they are ignorant but won't admit it—the vast majority of radiologists are very sharp cookies indeed.

The first theory is toxic peer review. Many institutions have this. A selection of your reports are judged against a standard. Now this isn't too bad in itself. It's an established quality method. But only if the standard is beyond approach, the judgement accurate and the consequences merely educational. Often they are nothing of the sort. Which has endless negative ramifications on reporting practice.

The second is that you usually only find out about your mistakes. You rarely find out if you were right. Faced with repeated negative feedback, it is easy to become dispirited and excessively cautious. Indeed, radiology is like playing golf in the dark. But you will have to wait until Rule #72 to explore the notion further.

Chapter 41
Rule #41 / / Radiologists Don't Wear Suede Shoes

Or brogues, open toed shoes or sandals. You'll know why once you grasp the concept of second-hand barium.

—

A radiologist wearing suede shoes is a fool. It indicates one of three scenarios. The most likely state of affairs is that they are an innocent noob, blissfully unaware of the hazards ahead. It is less likely that they a foppish diagnostic radiologist who keeps their footwear clean by deliberately eschewing patient contact. Least likely is that they don't give a stuff and just pulled on what was closest to hand as they set off for work.

The same is true of brogues, sandals, flip-flops and other open-toed shoes. All of these types of foot-wear suffer the same problem: they are ill-suited to liquid spills. And in the healthcare environment, fluid goes south all the time. I'm not particularly clumsy but if had a penny for every time I wiped the floor after I'd spilled something in the workplace, I'd have about £2.67.

The liquids are varied in nature and origin. Sometimes the fluid issues from a patient. Patients have a tendency to, well, leak a bit. It is part of being ill, you see. Most of the leakages are accidental. Having said that, sometimes I'm not 100% sure. I should point out that we don't encourage leaks and spills. Radiology is supposed to be a relatively civil speciality. It specifically lacks gore. We like it that way. Generally, we prefer our patients to have their body fluids in the expected places.

Blood occasionally make an appearance in the radiology department. If a radiologist manages to get blood on their shoes, it is also a fair indication that something went awry. Even in interventional radiology the amounts of house red outside of the intravascular space should be fairly minimal.

Other less pleasant body fluids show their face less often. If sputum, urine or faeces ends up on your shoes then you are probably doing something wrong. Particularly if the body fluids in question aren't yours.

In radiology, the majority of spills are boring and just involve contrast media. The commonest of which is the water-soluble iodine-based stuff. Iodine is used as it is quite cheap (they get it from seaweed) plus it is quite dense and blocks X-rays nicely. Considering the sheer volume that we get through every day, it is unsurprising when some of it makes a successful bid for freedom. It is unexciting; sticky and gloopy but non-staining and odorous-free. Warm water and gentle sponging is all you need for spills of iodinated contrast.

We still use a fair bit of barium, again, a dense material that shows up beautifully on an X-ray. We don't use as much as we used to, admittedly. You may remember from high school chemistry that water-soluble barium salts (acetate, carbonate, chloride, fluoride, hydroxide, nitrate, and sulphide) are highly toxic. Just five grams of barium chloride is enough to finish off a full-grown human. The good news is that we don't use any of those. We use barium sulphate, which is completely non-toxic. The bad news for your shoes is that is insoluble.

Insoluble compounds can obviously be wiped easily from smooth non-porous material. Spill a bit on the floor and it is no problem. Spill it onto patterned leather or cloth and you'll be scrubbing the sodding stuff out for weeks. Get it on suede and it is frankly buggered.

Even worse is second-hand barium. This isn't some odd recycling thing. This is barium has been inside someone else before obeying Newton's Laws of Gravity. Now we either put it in the top end or the bottom end. It can leak from either end. It isn't often spat. Again, you are probably doing something very wrong if barium is spat at you.

As I've previously mentioned, the barium enema is on its last legs, certainly in the UK at least. Radiologists of my age and older will remember barium enemas with a bittersweet memory. Yes, it was a happier and more innocent time. But having second hand barium drip onto your shoes was one of those things that I do not miss one bit.

To be honest, I'm surprised more patients didn't leak. For those of you unfamiliar with the process, a barium enema involves raising a 600 ml bag of barium sulphate suspension to 1 m. This gives an intense rectal pressure, in excess of 1 atmosphere. Thank the Lord for those with intact sphincters. But you wore the incorrect shoes to a barium list only once.

Many radiologists change into theatre clogs when performing procedures. The old-school wooden soled clogs are very much still alive and kicking but a padded plastic simulacrum is preferred by the medical masses. Think easy-to-clean version of Crocs. There are now a wide variety available. My favourite personalisation was a glamorous female colleague who opted for a pair of sparkly gold ones.

On that matter, the semiotics of shoes is fascinating. What you wear on your feet speaks volumes about you. Especially if you wear flesh-coloured nine-inch Louboutin heels. A semiologist can really go to town as everyone wears shoes. Not everyone sports a hat, glasses or jewellery. Not everyone has piercings or tattoos. Or hair.

The colour is emblematic. Gold or silver speaks of glamour and flamboyance. Red indicates power, lust, danger and a hint of madness. Black speaks of neutrality, brown of orthodoxy and white of puritanism. Green or purple, in my limited experience, is strong evidence of a personality disorder.

Dirty or scuffed shoes signal slovenliness. Impractical footwear signifies vanity whereas patent leather reveals a lack of it. Highly polished leather is a muted appeal for your approval. Sandals in the workplace intimate self-confidence and concern for the planet. Slip-ons denote a lack of both pretension and self-respect. Sports shoes or street shoes on a healthcare worker over the age of thirty is a sign that they need to grow up. Either that or they have arthritis.

The more that you think about it, the more of a minefield it is. The bottom line is that your footwear reveals more about you than you perhaps realise. Given that most people have a choice of what they put their feet into, you can now use this to your advantage. Unless you have size 14 feet and just have to buy anything that fits [FX—muffled sobbing, blows nose noisily].

Socks are also a lesser known window to the soul. In years gone by, a gentleman wouldn't wear coloured socks and a lady wouldn't need them. There is a marvellous passage in PG Wodehouse's *The Inimitable Jeeves* where Bertie calls for his "jolly purple" socks only for Jeeves to lug "them out of the drawer as if he were a vegetarian fishing a caterpillar out of a salad".

Socks are no longer an mundane item of clothing. For males, they are the new tie. Consider a lovely pair of shiny brogues. Then compared the pairing of a lambswool sock with a subtle stripe vs saggy white sports socks jaundiced with sweat. A world of difference I think you'll find.

Black socks take no imagination to wear. But they also reveal the same about you. White socks broadcast that your mother is probably still doing your shopping for you. Solid eye-catching colour socks scream your Alpha status. They are the pedal equivalent of carrying a large blunt object.

Eccentric and colourful socks can put people at their ease. Or turn their stomachs. Wear Star Wars socks on May 4th and you are in the same cadre as Justin Trudeau and his infamous 'sock diplomacy'. On the other hand, a pair of Homer Simpson socks will eradicate any suspicions that you are even slightly amusing. It is a fine balance.

Most doctors are utilitarian about their footwear and clothing. They'll wear something neutral and smart for the majority of their day, changing into scrubs and theatre clogs for potentially messy procedures. Some doctors wear this as their default work clothing. Or various bits of this, say, just a scrub top or the clogs but normal trousers or skirt. In these post-pandemic days, I expect more folk will do the same.

Scrubs and clogs may give the illusion of cleanliness but honestly are no more hygienic that normal clothes and shoes. But certain institutions insist their healthcare workers wear them. A lot don't have a strict uniform code. Certainly radiologists in the U.K. don't have this. So why wear them if you don't have to?

The simplest reason is that you don't have to wash or iron them. Individuals who wear scrubs through personal sloth also don't change them regularly. And then they tend not to launder them, merely peeling them off and flinging them into a corner. So if you see a pile of used scrubs in an office corner, you are in the presence of a slob.

There is also a slight macho thing too. The inference is that if you are wearing scrubs and clogs then you are someone who indulges in hard-core and gory procedures. If you are an interventional radiologist then you are doing this, just via pin-holes. On the flip side, if you are a diagnostic radiologist that habitually wears scrubs and clogs then it could be that you still like dressing up, pretending to be a surgeon. Which is a little sad. Either that or you really, really hate ironing shirts. Which I totally get.

Chapter 42
Rule #42 / / Never Investigate On The Day Of Discharge

Such tests always turn up something unexpected. It'll prove ultimately benign but will take a week to sort out.

—

A phenomenon of the last decade is the 'discharge-dependent' scan. I cannot abide it. The phrase makes me physically recoil, as if I've caught a sudden waft of rotten kipper. We are typically told that 'if Mrs Bloggs has a normal scan, she can go home'. It is a hollow and empty phrase. It is a bargaining chip used by inexperienced clinicians trying to get a non-urgent scan done super-quick.

On a cursory inspection, the concept holds water. Mrs Bloggs could leave the hospital if only the radiology department would extract the digit. Except on closer analysis, it doesn't work in 99% of cases. Scans can stop people coming into hospital, sure. There are three reasons that scans aren't stopping patients going home.

First, if Mrs Bloggs is ready to go home then so she should, toot sweet. You can guarantee that she won't want to stay. Being a hospital inpatient is extremely boring. If you are *compos mentis* you get cabin fever within a few days. Plus hospitals are expensive. At >£300 a day most hotels are cheaper and their food is infinitely better. Also hospitals are risky places to loiter. You are a sitting duck for hospital-acquired infections, not to mention DVTs and constipation.

Second, on the day of discharge, the illness 'journey' is nearing completion. Mrs Bloggs must be well or marching down the road to wellness. Therefore she has had all the requisite investigations, had appropriate therapy and at least started to make a recovery. *Ipso facto* she doesn't need any more scans. Or if she does, they certainly aren't part of her current treatment, are therefore non-urgent and shouldn't stop her from going home.

Third and most important is the negative investigational paradigm. You are doing the scan with the expectation that it will be normal. This is as opposed to attempting to prove your diagnosis by finding positive evidence. The usual excuse I hear is that clinicians want to 'rule out' or 'exclude' a particular diagnosis before

P. McCoubrie, *The Rules of Radiology*, https://doi.org/10.1007/978-3-030-65229-6_42

discharge. As we saw in Rule #33, this is absolute BS. No self-respecting radiologist allows scans on this basis.

Attempting to prove a diagnosis by 'ruling out' other diagnoses is completely illogical. It is seeking negative evidence, gathering evidence of absence. This rarely proves anything. A single piece of positive evidence can prove a point but it is much much harder to prove anything with negative evidence. You can infer very little about a diagnosis with only normal test results in front of you.

For example, say I suddenly smell the distinctive aroma of eucalyptus. I thoroughly search the room and find no koalas. I am therefore happy that a *Phascolarctos cinereus* masticating gum leaves is not the explanation. But that leaves me no wiser as to the source of the odour.

Under a negative paradigm you would confirm your diagnosis by seeking to disprove all other possibilities. As well as looking for antipodean arboreal marsupials I'd check my pot of Tiger Balm in the bathroom was intact then go into the street to smell the hair of passers-by just in case it was their shampoo. Clearly this is bonkers. Normal folk would spot the new air freshener on the mantelpiece and give it a confirmatory sniff.

The same is true about investigation of the ill person. You don't make a diagnosis by excluding all other possibilities. This is like using radiology as a club, bludgeoning a diagnosis to death. You use scans as a precision instrument to confirm a specific diagnosis. It is by far the quickest and most efficient method.

Hospitals aren't always such cold and logical places. They are stuffed with irrationalities and superstitious nonsense. For example, you'll never see anything labelled "13". There are no room 13s, cubicle 13s or ward 13s. It is 12b. Or they skip it completely, going from twelve straight to fourteen. I wish I was joking.

And just like actors will refer to Macbeth as the 'Scottish Play', hospital staff are superstitious about the word 'quiet'. You might describe slow trade as a lull, calm or tranquil. Anyone using the 'Q word' is hissed at for tempting fate. Say the Q word and the peaceful shift of your dreams becomes a screaming nightmare as a tsunami of work suddenly sweeps in.

Now I'm not a believer in fate. My destiny is not mapped in the stars. No supernatural being has it all planned out. But I would not have any medical investigations just before going on holiday, on the day before a long holiday weekend, or just prior to a major life event.

The fatalist would argue that you are just asking for an abnormal test. However I reason that you'll ruin the subsequent occasion by worrying about the result. Or if you get the results, then you can't take any action for several days. I can attest that is a singularly frustrating experience, particularly if the test is abnormal.

Of course Lady Luck plays no part in the accuracy of a test. It's function is unaffected by the time of day, day of the week and so forth. But it does seem that false positives crop up when you least want them to. Spurious abnormalities and borderline findings seem to occur at the most awkward times. Don't believe me? Have an x-ray on the morning of your wedding. Guaranteed borderline abnormal.

This isn't fate. It is because false positive rates are a complex statistical beast. If you are expecting a scan to be normal then most positive results are false positive.

It is because low prevalence lowers the positive predictive ability of the test. It is a statistical fact; I'm not making it up. It is why spurious positive findings are the only thing you find if you investigate on the day of discharge.

It isn't unusual for healthy people to have abnormal test results. Most tests have a normal range of measurements which is generally estimated to two standard deviations from the norm. Hence the normal range excludes the upper and lower 2.5%. Therefore 5% of the population will be labelled abnormal even if there is nothing wrong with them. This is no false positive test result; the test is perfectly accurate. It is just statistical bad luck that this particular individual lies outside a normal range.

Not only that but the more tests you do, the more likely that one will come back abnormal. If a person has twenty tests there is a sixty-six percent chance of one or more abnormal results. This isn't just numerical laboratory measurements such as blood counts but the more subjective radiological and pathological tests too. Given the 'supermarket requesting' model of modern clinical care, twenty tests would be the absolute minimum for most hospital admissions.

We also often find minor abnormalities of dubious significance. The term 'incidentaloma' was coined in 1982, originally to describe small adrenal lumps. It has since emerged that if you look hard enough at most organs then most of them contain little benign lumps. The problem is that they are difficult to distinguish from early cancers. So modern radiology brings with it an inevitable flurry of incidentalomas.

The next problem with borderline or spurious findings is that you have to somehow prove them to be innocuous. Perhaps you simply repeat the original test. You may need an appropriate specialist to officially pooh-pooh them. Further confirmatory testing may be needed. This takes time and inconvenience on behalf of the patient. If something invasive like a biopsy is required, it is not without discomfort or a degree of risk.

In 1972, Mercer Rang christened this process the 'Ulysses syndrome'. He described patients that underwent a 'long journey through the investigative arts and experience a number of adventures before reaching their point of departure once again', noting it was akin to Ulysses' twenty years of dramatic exploits on trying to return home after the Trojan war. Crucially he stated it was a benign phenomenon that carried a better prognosis that uninvestigated disease.

A more recent author disagreed. In 2003 Richard Heywood wrote a memorable personal view in the *BMJ* in which he coined the acronym VOMIT (Victim of Medical Imaging Technologies). He claimed that 'innocent pathology' on scans induced considerable worry and anxiety in patients and their families.

This 'acronym for our time' seemed to strike a chord; a flurry of letters were sent to the editor. Further facetious acronyms were suggested including: Brainless Application of Radiological Findings (BARF), Ominous Referrals for Dubious Unattested Radiographic Examinations (ORDURE) leading to suggestions for the setting up of the Campaign for Real Ailments (CAMRA).

It is isn't just radiological tests, it applies to all investigations that are highly sensitive yet not particularly specific. Any screening programme is exactly the same. The Prostate Specific Antigen (PSA) test for prostate cancer is sometimes referred to as 'Promoting Stress and Anxiety'. The tests themselves can be the problem. For example, there is a sweet irony that Breast Screening to detect cancer uses x-ray mammography which can itself cause cancer.

I hope you are now persuaded that investigating on the day of discharge is a very bad idea. It is logically flawed, causes the Ulysses syndrome induces VOMIT and stops patients from going home. That is why no-one gets a 'discharge-dependent' scan from me.

Chapter 43
Rule #43 / / Only Give Clinicians 15 Seconds

If they can't cut to the chase, help them. We haven't got all day. The longer the pre-amble, the lower the pre-test probability.

—

The goal of any professional is to be slick. I'm not talking showy or smarmy; most doctors don't see medicine as a performance art. A slick radiologist has polished professionalism. Tasks are discharged quickly and competently. Not only that, the skilful smoothness allows your actions to look effortless when, in reality, they are far from easy.

Appreciating this slickness only really comes from having had to learn it yourself. Most lay folk won't even notice. That is the point. If people notice what you are doing then you are not slick. In a top class restaurant, the waiters seemingly emerge from nowhere. With the best radiologists the needle is barely noticed and the procedure is over before you know it.

Slickness isn't being a robot either. You need more than ruthless efficiency of motion and deed. Slickness requires flexibility, adaptability and an ability to react quickly to when matters change, vary or don't follow the expected path. Slickness is remaining unruffled and smiling when things get difficult. Slickness is calmly delivering a good result even when things get distinctly sweaty.

Learning to be slick isn't just repetitive physical rehearsal, although this is important. It isn't innate physical dexterity either. Nimbleness can be learnt. The truth is that slickness involves a huge amount of knowledge. Most slickness is about rapid and complex decision making, based on a deep working knowledge of the task in hand.

Getting to be slick is a bit of a black box. You start out all bumbling and, an indeterminate amount time later, you are reasonably slick. But how is this achieved? The traditional approach to learning how to be slick is akin to a cook-book. You put together your ingredients methodically, follow an agreed recipe, stick to agreed timings and you get good results. Slickness comes from following the same steps over and over again.

This is how curricula work. It is how most instructional programs work. You deconstruct a task into smaller and easier to learn steps. Perform all the steps in order and a novice can reliably achieve reasonable results. Practice the recipe and you can produce consistently excellent results in a decent time. Except it doesn't really work like that in professional practice.

Healthcare isn't like a relaxed home kitchen. A cookbook gets you only so far. Ingredients are often missing, you frequently have half the time specified and the kitchen may be on fire. And even if you follow precisely the same steps you can get a completely different result. Furthermore, if your recipe goes wrong, people can die.

Becoming a master of your art involves knowing the recipe backwards, being able to skilfully perform each step blindfold and possibly improving on the original. It also entails knowing endless variations of ingredients, different tools that can be employed, safe shortcuts, pitfalls and how to bail yourself out when it goes wrong. It is why learning the recipe is only the first step on a long journey.

The traditional model of radiology training focuses almost exclusively on 3 topics:- image interpretation, communication of the findings and procedural skill. And rightly so. You'd be bloody useless unless you master these three aspects. The only problem is that time and motion studies show that radiologists only spend roughly half their time doing this. The other half is largely the production and ingestion of coffee as well as a few piffling quanta of other professional activities.

These activities unrelated to ritualised caffeine abuse can be loosely clustered as 'professional skills'. Sometimes called non-technical skills, they rarely appear on the curriculum and if they do, usually as an after-thought, tacked on to appease the politically correct brigade. I've long held that they are as important as interpretational and procedural skill. In fact, they cannot be thought of as distinct. They are integral to professionalism.

I recently stood up at a national conference to talk about this. Partly for a cheap laugh, I said a radiologist is like a meat pie. The crust is the professional outer that protects and enhances the inner human. A decent meat pie needs a hot-water crust. This is a balance of three ingredients. In this model, hot water is procedural skill, flour is interpretational skill and lard is professional skills that binds it together. The filling is you: hopefully a healthy and happy individual.

The best pies have both a toothsome crust and a well-seasoned and juicy filling. If you are all crust and no filling then you are an empty soulless individual, skilled but a husk of your former self, possibly burntout. If you are all filling and no crust then you are undoubtedly lovely but talentless and highly vulnerable.

You may not be aware of the concept of professional skills or non-technical skills. They are individual cognitive skills and social behaviours, distinct from personality. In the airline industry they are called Crew Resource Management. Of the six key tenets of professional skills the most important for a radiologist are communication, decision-making, situational awareness and teamwork. They all sound like common sense stuff but each is a discrete field of scientific endeavour with a voluminous literature and heaps of evidence about best practice.

Professional skills are common to every profession but more important to those whose job carries risk. So, if you are a check-out operator, you probably don't give two stuffs about professional skills and rightly so. If you are an airline pilot or interventional radiologist and literally have to make life and death decisions, professional skills are crucial to get right.

You may think that a jobbing diagnostic radiologist wouldn't need an explicit understanding of professional skills. Their job involves few crises except, perhaps, when the departmental coffee machine goes on the blink. It is a mistake to think professional skills are only needed in a crisis. We all use them. And when things go wrong, it usually comes down to a failure of professional skills. Poor communication is one of the most frequent causes of medical error.

It follows that all radiologists should be expert communicators. We are no different to any other doctor in that respect. However this Rule contradicts conventional teaching. We are taught to let patients tell their story and not interrupt them. Doctors frequently don't do this but that is a separate story.

Time invested in communication before a scan is time well spent. The patient gets the right scan at the right time and the clinical question is answered. It is important to weed out unwarranted scans. No one wants to join in on a diagnostic fishing trip, where the investigation rod is cast hither and thither. No one wants to be part of a scatter-gun approach, where the patient is bombarded by tests in the vain hope that something will turn up.

There is a trade-off. You need a reasonable amount of information to answer the question. But a flood of information helps only marginally more than a modest amount. So you need a balance. Long enough to glean the basics but not a moment too long.

It is for this reason that I explicitly advocate closing down a clinician fifteen seconds into their spiel. This is explicitly during a consultation. Don't do this during a social call. That would be weird. Obviously do it tactfully and politely. You can use non-verbal methods too. This said, I would advocate against placing a hand over their mouth. Not least because there is a chance of biting, especially from surgeons.

Fifteen seconds is plenty of time. You can describe everything a radiologist needs to know in far less. Admittedly this needs a certain amount of marshalling of thoughts and succinctness. But distilling a brief summary of the clinical problem and what they want of you is, if you think about it, easily achievable.

Generally the younger the clinician, the longer the spiel. Also the less macho the speciality, the longer the spiel. A young psychiatrist will typically deliver a protracted monologue but a senior surgeon pops their head around the door, grunts, "Pancreatitis; CT", lobs a request form at us and scarpers.

It is also true that the longer the initial pitch, the less likely we are to find anything. A Shakespearian soliloquy means the scan will definitely be normal. A terse sentence or two guarantees an absolute car-crash of a scan.

A big part of being a clinician is being slick at referrals and consultations. Nobody wants a rambling story that ends with, "Oops, sorry, wrong patient". We want, "Mrs Bloggs is day 6 of acute pancreatitis, please can we have a CT to assess its severity?".

Giving unexpurgated details about patients may feel like good practice but paradoxically it impedes good patient care. It slows you down. Slow means you don't see the next patient quickly. Care given at a glacial pace is rarely appropriate in a modern hospital. Young doctors need to learn and radiologists should be there to help them. A radiologist cutting off a circumlocutory clinician is actually delivering valuable CPD.

Clinicians need to know that we appreciate brevity. In fact, everyone wants concision. Everyone is busy. Quick but crap is in no one's best interests. Good but slow means no one gets their work done. Slickness, after all, is a combination of good and quick. Slickness is the unofficial aim of post-graduate training.

Chapter 44
Rule #44 / / You Can Never Know Too Much Anatomy

The more anatomy you know, the better the radiologist you become. It's the only thing you learn at medical school that won't have changed by the time you retire.

—

Anatomy is to radiology as geography to history; it describes the scene of action. Surgeons get this. Pathologists too. They appreciate that it is difficult to properly understand disease without understanding what normal looks like. Pathologists are like old-school car mechanics, looking at the disassembled parts, sucking through their teeth. Radiologists diagnose the problems non-invasively, like modern car mechanics who just plug the car into a computer. Surgeons claim that operating is like fixing the engine whilst it is running. Whereas Physicians just sniff the exhaust pipe and add tincture of foxglove to the petrol.

Physicians have little need of detailed anatomy. They don't need to see inside people to make a diagnosis. Their anatomical knowledge withers away. In fact, they seem to know so little that I suspect the Membership of the Royal College of Physicians' admission ceremony involves ablation of a certain portion of the brain. This disparity in knowledge is why a radiologist can easily feel superior to a physician.

It is a truism that one cannot be a decent radiologist without being a decent anatomist. But radiology is much more than just applied anatomy. The difference between an anatomist and a radiologist is simple. The anatomist is like a taxi driver who knows all the narrowest and most distant streets. A radiologist knows all the streets but also knows the houses and what is going on inside them.

In that respect, radiologists have also been compared to estate agents. Our jobs are perfect for the inquisitive sort. An estate agent gets to have a good nosy around other people's houses; a radiologist gets to have a good nosy around other people's innards. Except estate agents aren't asked to diagnose blocked drains. Nor are they called at 2am when a pipe blows and there is blood everywhere.

P. McCoubrie, *The Rules of Radiology*, https://doi.org/10.1007/978-3-030-65229-6_44

It is a privilege to visually rummage around a patient's giblets. I admit to getting slightly excited about anatomy in a way that the average lay person wouldn't understand. Sometimes it gets the better of me when I unconsciously mumble "beautiful" after having seen the pancreas very clearly on ultrasound. I've also had to explain myself to a patient when I described her gallbladder as "exquisite", causing her to laugh out loud. Radiologists will get this professional glee; others are left scratching their head.

Anatomy is the lingua franca of the body. Well, almost. The *Terminologica Anatomica* lists over 7000 anatomical structures in the human body in both English and Latin (either is acceptable). Anatomists talk in a slightly different dialect to radiologists. For example, we talk about the duodenum having parts one to four, they talk about the superior, descending, horizontal, and the ascending parts. They also talk mysteriously about a hidden part. But they should know better. You can't hide anything from a radiologist - they can see right through you.

Anatomy has been around for much longer than radiology. Galen's work in the second century AD dominated anatomical thinking for more than 1300 years until 1543 when Vesalius published *De humani corporis fabrica*. Vesalius had the advantage that his work was based on actual dissection of humans rather than on theory and supposition. Even then Galenian thinking dominated. William Harvey's 1628 *de Motu Cordis* on circulation of the blood took over twenty years to be accepted.

And so whilst anatomical enlightenment took centuries, radiology has opened new ways of seeing the human body in it's comparatively brief existence. No longer is the study of anatomy like learning from the display in a butchers shop window. Although in fairness, being a radiologist does change the way that you view cuts of meat. I look at pork chops quite differently these days. Plus I have new-found respect for the psoas muscle: lamb, pork or beef fillets are solely comprised of this muscle.

Most health professionals study anatomy to some degree. Medics study it in a little more detail than most. Maybe too much detail, to be honest. From anatomy's heyday in Victorian times it has been taught without much consideration for practical application. For example, medical students have long been taught the intricacies of the brachial plexus, a particular knot of nerves that control arm and shoulder movement. Sadly this knowledge is utterly superfluous. No one needs to know how such millimetre-thin nerves interconnect. Well, maybe ten or twenty people in the whole world at the most.

Medical school teaching that is irrelevant is dangerous as it dilutes the relevant stuff and overloads the student. Depressingly, it's nothing new. In 1863 the UK's General Medical Council raised a concern about the tendency of 'overloading of the curriculum of education … followed by results injurious to the student'. I could cite many similar references in the intervening 160 years.

British author and doctor Somerset Maugham also wrote about this over a century ago. In his *bildungsroman* 'Of Human Bondage' his first medical school lecturer paraphrased Tennyson:

"You will have to learn many tedious things," he finished, with an indulgent smile, "which you will forget the moment you have passed your final examination, but in anatomy it is better to have learned and lost than never to have learned at all".

Nearly a century later, students are still cramming for exams then promptly forgetting everything. There are many reasons for bloated curricula. Sometimes teaching can be paradoxically too up to date. There have always been fashions and trends in medical education. Sir Robert Hutchison said in 1925, "We must not inseminate the virgin minds of the young with the tares of our own fads… It is always well, before handing the cup of knowledge to the young, to wait until the froth has settled."

He was largely ignored. In 1977 Hugh Dudley wrote, "Virtually anything that is new will be popular at the time of its introduction and for a few years thereafter because the medical course is so dull … [but] At least 75% of innovations will have a half-life of less than five years."

Yes, he was a curmudgeon but the ordering effect is very real. This is where the most recently adopted approach, with the most associated enthusiasm, always wins. This can lead to an 'educational purgatory' of constant curriculum change. Constant innovation edges out older subjects and brings cries of 'dumbing down' from grey-haired doctors in grey suits. Despite all this, anatomical training is still there, firmly fixed in the first year of medical school training.

Medical school trains you to be a new doctor but is poor preparation for being a new radiologist. Bizarrely radiology barely appears on medical school curricula. Radiology is now one of the biggest departments in the hospital yet has no academic department in many UK medical schools. There are twice as many radiologists as pathologists in the UK yet pathologists still get plenty of student bum-seat/ hours (the currency of curriculum time).

Young radiologists have to learn their anatomy almost from scratch. This is partly because important anatomy has been forgotten the alongside irrelevance of the roots and cords of the brachial plexus. Undergraduate educational failings aren't everything though. Even ex-surgeons starting in radiology still have a hill to climb. This is because anatomy in radiology has a different slant. It all visual rather than visceral. It is also different in format; either projectional if based on a x-ray or cross-sectional. It isn't just axial like a bacon slice either. Any and all anatomical planes are used.

Radiological anatomy is very much the first stage of radiological training, certainly in the UK. The first FRCR anatomy exam in the UK is sat after just six months of training. I was a Royal College anatomy examiner for seven years and it gave me numerous insights into radiological anatomy. Did you know, for example, that every year at least one young radiologist will confidently label an arrowed structure in the female pelvis as the 'vagine'?

Young radiologists are often overcome with the amount they have to learn. I remember starting my training and looking up in despair at the mountain of knowledge that I had to climb. Nowadays I try to allay my young charges by describing the five stages of radiology training. The first step is to recognise what is normal. The second step is to recognise what is abnormal. The third step is know what the abnormality is. The fourth step is to know it's significance. The fifth step is to communicate this clearly.

Each step takes roughly one year and it is no surprise that radiology training is five years long in many countries. It is also why radiology registrars start to become useful in their third year. I explain to newbie radiologists that it will take them at least six months to find the adrenal glands on CT. And then another four years to ignore all the tiny incidental lumps they find.

When all is said and done, anatomy is the bedrock on which the radiology house is built. Just like the wise builder in the Bible (Matthew 7:24–27), a wise radiologist is glad of the investment in solid foundations when the rains, floods and winds of professional practice beat against them and yet they stand firm. A foolish radiologist that knows little anatomy is building their career on sand. The lightest of inclement weather is bad news for those with poor foundations.

Chapter 45
Rule #45 / / Be Careful With "Limited" Or "Quick" Studies

Guaranteed you'll miss the cancer. Better off doing the full Monty or nothing at all.

—

There is a world of difference between a radiologist truncating a study and the patient doing so. If a patient signals that they want a radiological procedure to stop, it stops. Saying 'stop' is withdrawing consent to proceed. Thus not stopping is committing assault. These are the facts. Having control over what others do to your body is an inviolable human right. Even if the radiologist is totally convinced they are doing the right thing, they must down tools. Even if the goal of the procedure was in touching distance, it must remain unattained.

Patient choice wasn't always taken so seriously. It used to be quite acceptable to persuade patients to either have a procedure or not have it, as the radiologist felt appropriate. The 'doctor knows best' was an accepted societal norm. This paternalistic model has been rightly rejected. Even if the doctor feels they know best, they have to acquiesce to the absolute right of individuals to make choices over their body. Even if the choices seem completely irrational, radiologists are legally obliged to accept those choices. However, if patient lacks mental capacity then that is legally different (and much more complex).

The correct moral stance is to provide the patient with information to allow them to make an informed decision. Easy peasy, you might think. Wrong. It is horrendously difficult to do this well. First you have to explain complicated medical matters to a frightened and potentially vulnerable patient. Second, you have to explain risks and benefits in a way they can understand. Last, you have to guide them through their choices in an unbiased and calm manner. To do this effectively is very hard. To do this badly is very easy.

Of course there is a moral obligation to do no harm (see Rule #28). A patient may want a scan or procedure but the radiologist can refuse to do it if they think it might cause harm. Also, a radiologist can refuse to do a procedure if they think it will not help the patient. A clinician may jump up and down as much as they want but radiologists are not beholden to the tantrums of others. Futility is an important concept in radiology, particularly in the frail elderly, and will be discussed more fully in Rules #59 and #64.

If I am honest, the text above could be straight out of a standard medical ethics textbook. It isn't, of course. I may be derivative but I'm not a plagiarist. But, as ever, there are grey areas in professional practice. There are, if you look carefully, pitfalls everywhere. I'll detail a few examples.

Is it OK to reassure a nervous patient? (Fig. 45.1) They understand the risks but are just worried. A compassionate radiologist might squeeze their hand, look them in the eye and reassure them that they are in the best hands. But you could argue this is unethical as reassurances are a form of coercion. You might not be intending to but it is an easy trap to fall into.

Another example is what constitutes withdrawal of consent during a procedure. Obviously the patient screaming, "For the love of God, please stop!" is not exactly a moral conundrum. But if a patient squawks as your needle hits a spot that the local anaesthetic hasn't quite reached, causing them to levitate transiently off the table, is this a time to check you still have consent? Or do you apologise, infiltrate a touch more lidocaine and carry on?

A last example is where the radiologist feels uncomfortable in doing a procedure but is persuaded by the clinician. Clinicians browbeat radiologists to varying

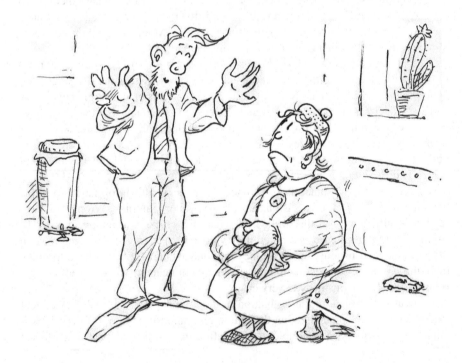

Fig. 45.1 Is it OK to reassure a nervous patient?

degrees. Key phrases to watch out for are, "Could you give a quick mouthful of barium to...", "I know your list is full but could you just...", "I have a rather interesting patient...". These are the polite ways radiologist have their arms twisted. Emotive pleas are also quite common. A colleague just the other weekend had a clinician plead, "But... but...it's a child we are talking about".

The dilemma is exacerbated when the radiologist finds that the description of the patient bears no resemblance to that which was promised. The promised lump cannot be found and the patient adds, "Yes, the doctor said they couldn't feel it either". The 'cooperative patient' arrives wild-eyed, delirious, with a single upper incisor. The allegedly 'previously fit and well' patient turns out to be quadriplegic; well, they would have been before the bilateral leg amputation. Does the radiologist pull the plug or carry on regardless?

This is why radiologists may sometimes truncate or abbreviate a procedure. This is different from the various ways to improve a scan that was discussed in Rule #34. This is taking shortcuts or omission of whole sections of a procedure out of concern for the patient. The radiologist deliberately curtails the study. This is for a variety of reasons.

This could be self-preservation. Patients can be pugnacious due to disease. Both dementia and delirium can induce a previously benign and saintly granny to have a pop at a stranger. It is not granny's fault, bless her wispy white curls. But don't underestimate the punch that a delirious octogenarian can pack. If the patient is hostile but neither demented nor delirious then they get short shrift. We have no time for that nonsense.

Radiologists often shorten a procedure because the patient is looking distinctly peaky at the outset. The patient arrives ill and the radiologist doesn't want to make things worse. Or the patient takes a turn for the worse mid-procedure. Either way, it is in everyone's best interests if the procedure is done and dusted in record time. The radiology department is ironically not the best place to fall mild-moderately ill. We don't have the staff or equipment for that. Have a cardiac arrest and we'll sort you out. But short of that you'd be better off anywhere else.

Just occasionally, the radiologist truncates a scan or procedure out of kindness. They may know the patient well and want to cause as little discomfort as possible. The patient may be disabled, immobile or already in pain and the radiologist doesn't want to add to their troubles. This is a balance. Obviously a heartless monster will ignore the patient's comfort in the quest for a perfecttechnical outcome. And a complete softie will settle for anequivocal outcome for fear of causing suffering. The correct balance is of course somewhere in the middle. As a general rule, if a radiologist has to be cruel to be kind then they should be kind whilst being cruel. If you catch my drift.

It is inexcusable to truncate a study purely because you are rushing. A good radiologist never rushes (see Rule #21). They either have time to do a procedure properly or they don't. And if they don't but it is urgent, then they either make time or find someone who has time. It is odd that urgent studies crop up at the least opportune time. We used to call these 'Crackerjack referrals', named after the

British kids TV programme whose opening tag line was "It's Friday, it's five to five and it's… Crackerjack!".

As we saw in Rule #9, finding time for an extra scan or other procedure is a delicate balance. If you are the radiologist who always makes time, always goes the extra mile and ends up staying late every night, then you are being exploited. On the flip side, I've recently heard of a radiologist that walks out precisely at five pm everyday, irrespective of who or what is still waiting to be done. Their job plan says they finish at five pm and so they jolly well finish at five pm. Except it isn't exactly endearing to colleagues or the patient, is it?

Of course the answer to finding time for urgent procedures is not staying late, working faster, or overloading muggins. This is like trying to pour a quart into a pint pot. It never works and you end up with unwanted fluids everywhere. The answer is designing a system that firstly has adequate time to get everything done without rushing and has capacity for unplanned urgent work.

Rushing a radiological procedure is no problem ninety-five percent of the time. Most of the scans we do are normal. Most procedures are uncomplicated. It isn't superstition or fatalistic to know that things that rushing is associated with a greater chance of going hideously wrong. No one would deliberately set out to knowingly increase the risk to a patient. So a radiologist must be calm and ignore external time pressures. When they are beginning a study, they should enter a zen-like state, put their watch aside and not look at the clock. The radiologist should give the procedure their full and undivided attention and thereby do a thorough job.

To help them focus, radiologists should imagine every patient is the Prime Minister. Actually, ignore that. This current one isn't exactly universally popular. Nor was the last. I wouldn't want to be known as the radiologist who incited others to assault their patients mid-procedure.

Chapter 46
Rule #46 / / Image Quality Is Up To The Radiologist

Image noise, coverage, adequacy of position and so on are all dictated by what you are willing to accept, not by what was produced.

—

You might think that this is an odd topic to include in the Rules; a dry technical matter amidst juicy clinical issues. Image quality is, I will admit, not particularly sexy. It isn't terribly controversial. Nor is it funny. In fact, as a subject, it is as dry as old bones. Very old bones that have been in a desert. Then fossilised.

But discuss it we must. Image quality is one of the cornerstones of radiology. To discuss radiology without an exposition on image quality would be like drinking gin without tonic; unthinkably tragic, verging on the barbaric.

Radiologists are quietly obsessed with image quality. There is nothing difficult about the concept at all. The better the image, the easier the diagnosis is. That's it. They don't go on about it; there is usually nothing to discuss. The only times that discussion occurs is either (i) a God-awful image has been submitted for reporting and the radiologist wants to know what went wrong, or (ii) a discussion about the fine line between torturing a patient and getting diagnostic images.

Image quality can become a partisan issue. A particular radiology department or even an individual radiologist can become renowned for the quality of certain studies. Most often because their images are particularly good but occasionally because they are infamously terrible. Acquisition of certain scanners can induce either jealousy or pity from other hospitals, depending on what has been bought.

Some hospitals regularly update and replace their older scanners. Others drag their heels, replacing them only when they can no longer be serviced. Some radiology departments are always building an extension for an additional scanner to cope with demand. Others just flog the existing kit harder.

You might think new scanners are always better and building work is a healthy sign. You might also think that it is depressing to work surrounded by ageing kit. But it isn't as simple as that. Old scanners represent good value for money,

P. McCoubrie, *The Rules of Radiology*, https://doi.org/10.1007/978-3-030-65229-6_46

important in these straitened times. Old scanners are simpler and have known foibles; new ones are complex and of uncertain reliability. Plus everyone moans for at least six months whilst learning how to use a new machine, emphasising how great the old one was.

Attitudes towards scanners vary widely elsewhere in the hospital. Heavy users of the radiology department, such as surgeons and oncologists, understand the need for decent kit. Others are less forgiving, seeing the radiology department as a financial vacuum that relentlessly hoovers money for new 'toys'. By the way, any self-respecting radiologist should never allow a scanner to be called a 'toy'. Toys are for children; this is a lightly veiled insult.

Making and selling scanners is a cut-throat business. The pace of technological development is dizzying. If a manufacturer takes their foot off the research and development pedal then they soon lose market position. Companies come and go, subsumed by one another seemingly on an annular basis. For example, we had a Marconi Mx8000 CT scanner which was rumoured to be rebranded Elscint technology although Picker were involved somewhere. Then Marconi was bought by Philips.

This obsession with ever improving image quality can only be good. Otherwise radiologists would be still guessing at the significance of smeared blotches of barely distinguishable grey. That said, the entire field of nuclear medicine imaging is exactly this. It isn't called 'Unclear Medicine' for nothing. The stuff they give to their patients? 'I-suppose-otopes'.

I actually find the whole field of nuclear medicine rather (wait for it) scintillating. And with that, I've told you three-quarters of the nuclear medicine jokes in existence. The last one is:- How do you get into the Nuclear Medicine department? Say 'Open Sestamibi'. There are no other Nuclear Medicine jokes. None.

Anyway. All radiologists learn the underlying science of image quality as part of their training. They are inculcated with importance of good images very early. In the UK this happens in the first six months when they learn about the Lamor frequency, Fourier half-transforms, and Aristotelian metaphysics. Actually, maybe not the last one. I forget. It was a long time ago.

Many then sit a famously tough exam full of hard science. In the UK it is the first FRCR Physics exam. Once they have passed it, they ceremoniously burn their revision notes and books, dance around the resultant fire, singing Hallelujah. Then promptly forget it all.

Learning how to be a radiologist by teaching raw basic science is a bit like learning to drive a car by first teaching how the engine works. Quite pointless really. I've been driving a car for over thirty years quite effectively. Yet I have absolutely no idea what a carburettor does. I think I did once but have forgotten. The same is true of 95% of medical physics that I crammed over twenty years ago.

When radiologists look at an image they not thinking about filtered back projection or the minutiae of the fast-spin echo technique. They are usually thinking 'What the hell is that blurry blob?' and musing on how acceptable it would be to close down the whole study and leave it for some other poor sap to report.

Surely, I hear you ask, you don't have to puzzle over blurry blobs anymore? With all the technical advances and whatnot, isn't it all automated or something? Or at least aren't modern radiology machines soooo much better than the old ones? Yes but no. The machines are tremendously complex but don't mistake advanced technology with magic. Generating radiological images of consistently good quality still requires a skilled touch.

There are three key ingredients to the generation of every radiological image:

- the machine you use
- the person using it
- the patient being examined

All three are infinite variables so you get unending variation. The skill comes in the person tailoring the machine to the individual patient.

It isn't always possible to get a textbook image. It isn't normally the fault of the machine, working within their tolerances and constrained by the laws of physics (but can have glitches). It isn't normally the fault of the radiographer, they too are using all their knowledge and experience (but can have an off day). It isn't normally the fault of the patient, they are trying to adopt the required position and hold still (but can be too ill or confused to do so).

Now. A minor excursion into technical matters. The best images are high resolution images that are motion-free. The glossy brochures of the multimillion dollar medical imaging industry are full of improbably sharp images. These are like catnip for radiologists. But we've had insanely detailed images for over 100 years. A standard chest X-ray film is approximately 150 gigapixels. Modern digital detectors still cannot match film in this respect.

Motion of the subject is nearly always bad because it causes blurring. Unless it is the motion that is being specifically looked at, say, calculating aspects of heart contraction or how the giblets writhe and contract (don't laugh - it's a thing, honest). Hence radiologists and other allied professionals have come up with a myriad of motion freezing techniques. The simplest is barked out a million times a day across the globe, "Breath in and hold your breath!".

There are two related technical issues I need to discuss, crucial for a good image. They are contrast and noise. Contrast and noise affect the ability to distinguish one blob from another because it is a different shade of grey. They are complex concepts - I will discuss contrast in more detail in Rule #48. Suffice it to say that contrast is good and radiologists would like as much of it as possible please. And image noise, or fuzziness, is bad. Radiologists would like as little as possible of that please.

The individuals that obtain ninety-nine percent of radiological images are radiographers, often called 'x-ray technicians' in other parts of the world. They spend a three year degree learning how to produce the best images possible. I must pay tribute to the art and skill of my radiographic colleagues. This isn't a faux devotion in an attempt to curry favour. Well, maybe a smidge.

Radiologists should always be kind to radiographers. On no account must you ever, ever, ever say to a radiographer something along the lines of, "Oh, are you the one that pushes the buttons?". This is a deathly insult. It is like asking a nurse if they wipe bottoms or calling an orthopaedic surgeon a glorified carpenter. Actually, that last one isn't too far off.

There are professional boundaries of responsibility. The responsibility of the person capturing the images stops after they've captured it and sent it for reporting. The person looking at the image has to then be able to make a diagnosis. If the image is poor then it might have to be repeated. As it is normally the radiographer acquiring the images and the radiologist looking at them, then the radiologist has to decide if the images are up to scratch.

For this reason radiologists are most often the arbiters of image quality. This is an important role of a radiologist. High standards are in everyone's best interest. If a radiologist permits poor quality images, they are inadvertently encouraging sloppiness. The standard that you walk past is the standard you accept. Which we'll look at more in Rule #90.

Chapter 47
Rule #47 / / It Is Never A Chordoma

Rare presentation of a common disease is commoner than common presentation of a rare disease. That classical rare bone lesion will turn out to be just another bone met.

—

In my younger days I was hungry for work. Eager to grow and learn as a young consultant, I would grab any scan that I thought was vaguely in my remit. The more esoteric and the more niche the scan, the more it got my radiological juices flowing. I wanted to develop depth of expertise as well as breadth. The best way, I reasoned, was to tackle difficult cases and learn from them. It still isn't a bad way to learn, actually.

However, this lead me to make a memorable mistake. I was looking at a 10 cm rounded mass eroding a poor soul's sacrum. It had been picked up on CT as the cause for their pain and I was looking at the MRI to try and help decide what it was. It was obviously a tumour of some sort but could any diagnostic clues be gained before it yielded it's secrets to a judicious 18G biopsy needle?

If you look up 'sacrum' in the Big Book of Radiology (Oh how I wish there was just the one), you won't find many entries. Not much happens in the sacrum, a stolid lump of bone at the bottom of the spine. Like any bone, it can be fractured. Sacral fractures are a miserable affair; either indicating you've torn your pelvis apart in some horrendous accident or it's cracked as your bones are paper-thin. But in the index of aforesaid tome, you'll find an alluring and mysterious entry 'sacro-coccygeal chordoma'.

I'd vaguely been aware of the diagnosis but never seen one. They are rare but the commonest primary tumour of the sacrum. The pictures looked exactly like the lesion in front of me. In fact, the more textbook cases I looked at, the more convinced I became: it was identical in all ways. I showed it to a colleague who agreed. So I reported it as 'typical features of a sacrococcygeal chordoma' and off I toddled, feeling warm inside.

© The Author(s), under exclusive license to Springer Nature Switzerland AG 2021
P. McCoubrie, *The Rules of Radiology*, https://doi.org/10.1007/978-3-030-65229-6_47

A few weeks later, I had word from colleague who had biopsied it that it was not a chordoma but an adenocarcinoma, probably a metastasis and, "Oh, didn't they tell you that she had a rectal cancer treated 2 years ago?", to which I answered, through gritted teeth, "No, they bloody well didn't". It is easy to blame others but you might have thought a previous history of malignancy in an organ only 2 cm away would have been relevant.

Anyway, I'm not telling you this story to induce sympathy or as a confession. I tell it as an illustration of a specific error of reasoning that is fairly common amongst radiologists. Interestingly radiologists aren't explicitly taught how to think. Philosophy and logic aren't on the curriculum. If you asked most radiologists about David Hume and the problems of inductive reasoning, I guarantee you'd be met with a blank-eyed stare.

In Rule #33 I semi-randomly introduced the phrase 'probabilistic hypothetico-deductive reasoning'. You might not be familiar with this being the basis of the clinical method. Let me explain. Diagnoses are very rarely 100% black or white. With the possible exception of a broken leg. Anyway, they are proposed or presented as a working hypothesis. The hypothesis is proved or refuted based on logical reasoning. This logic is informed by evidence from the patient's history, examination findings and test results.

Deductive reasoning is the historic method of putting this together into a water-tight case. So, in this case, the argument goes: (1) the patient had a large soft tissue mass in the sacrum; (2) large soft tissue masses are very likely to be malignant. Therefore, this patient's mass is very likely to be malignant. So long as the statements are true, deductive reasoning is risk-free.

Except most diagnoses don't lend themselves to deductive reasoning. Hard and fast evidence is often lacking. Or at least they don't move you forward very far. In reality, we usually start with a premise about a particular patient and attempt to make a generalisation. This is inductive reasoning. Because it involves probability, it is inherently risky.

So the inductive argument goes: The patient had a large soft tissue mass in the sacrum. Chordoma is a cause of large soft tissue mass in the sacrum. Therefore this patient has a chordoma. Well, not necessarily. The patient *could have* a chordoma. Inductive reasoning only works if you use probability arguments. And even then, as Hume himself observed, 'What *ought* to be cannot always be deduced from what *is*'.

If you think about it, this isn't what radiologists actually do in practice. They do a thing called 'abductive reasoning', a concept first proposed by Charles Sanders Peirce in the late 1800s. It is a blend of the two. This entails using what hard evidence you have to deduce the facts as far as you can and then you make a best guess through inductive reasoning thereafter.

The best guess or abduction is a pragmatic one. It is the simplest explanation that fits all the evidence available, otherwise known as Occam's Razor. William of Occam was a twelfth century English friar who might be horrified to hear this reduced to the KISS principle (Keep It Simple, Stupid). Abduction isn't perfect but is intended to give the most plausible diagnosis.

If you are still not completely clear then the best example of abductive reasoning is the Duck Test. This goes, "If it looks like a duck, swims like a duck, quacks like a duck, then it probably is a duck". Or as Douglas Adams parodied, "we have to at least consider the possibility that we have a small aquatic bird of the family *Anatidae* on our hands".

Back to my chordoma misdiagnosis, where my abductive reasoning was faulty. On this occasion it is clear that I made an error of probabilistic judgement. I saw a lump in the sacrum and thought it was a chordoma. So where did I go wrong? It wasn't a snap intuitive judgement, I really thought long and hard about it. I even asked a colleague.

The colleague fell into the specific error of 'confirmation bias'. This is where someone else's judgement affects your thinking. You are much more likely to agree with a colleague. It's a social behaviour. It is also why radiologists should always look at an image unburdened by what anyone else thinks, explicitly avoiding this bias.

My error of judgement was clear. Just like any human, I am prone to bias when working out clinical probabilities. Nobel Prize winner Daniel Kahneman has written about these, as we discussed in Rule #28. This particular howler was a special blend of three biases:

- First and foremost; availability bias. This is the bias that comes from the immediacy of recent events. For example, if you buy a new blue car, suddenly you notice every other person seems to have a blue car. I'd just read up on chordomas so I was primed to diagnose one.
- Second, is representativeness bias. This is the bias where you overestimate the probability of an event. For example, any article on sacral tumours will clearly state that the most common sacral tumours are metastases. But this fact is buried on page seven as metastases are not very sexy. Primary tumours like chordomas are much more exotic, hence they appear on page one despite being distinctly uncommon.
- Third is anchoring and adjusting bias. In medicine this is simply determining how likely the diagnosis is before and after a test. This is what doctors do every day. If your knowledge is expert level, you aren't affected by these biases much. However, if you are not an expert, you will be inaccurate at judging the likelihood of the diagnosis before or after the test. Fifteen years ago I most certainly was not an expert on sacral tumours. In the interim, I've seen hundreds of sacral tumours. All were metastases and not one single chordoma.

You may be left feeling completely bereft of any confidence in radiologists. I understand. 'Best guesses' don't inspire confidence do they? Acknowledging that multiple sources of bias affect even educated and intelligent people might further reduce your confidence. But do note that, despite its flaws, diagnostic reasoning currently outstrips anything computers can offer and works well in the majority of cases.

Where there is human illness, there will always be uncertainty. Where there is uncertainty, we quantify it into probability. Very precise probabilities can be given in many clinical scenarios, according to the proponents of evidence-based medicine. But textbook probabilities often don't reflect real-world scenarios. Clinical reasoning is an imperfect science because it is extrapolating from textbooks to the scenario in front of you. The diagnostic abilities of a radiologist are therefore the art and science of making calculated bets and educated guesses. There. I said it.

This is why a radiologist has to know loads (Rule #39). Knowing loads leads to accurate estimates of probability. Good use of probability leads to better decision making, resulting in better outcomes. The ability to accurately estimate probability is the hallmark of a good radiologist. This is partly why a radiologist has to know about esoteric diagnoses. But you will have to read Rule #52 to find out more.

Chapter 48
Rule #48 / / Reporting Rooms Should Be Pitch Black

If you report with the lights on, you are letting the entire profession down. Reporting in a dark room is for logical visual reasons but it also handily disorientates those who trespass.

—

This Rule is actually a lie, a shameless headline-grab. Reporting rooms should be dark, that much is true. But not pitch black. The ambient lighting should be as bright as the computer monitor. The reason is simple. Your eyes get tired if you have to constantly readjust as your vision moves from dark surroundings to bright screen and back again.

Now you may be thinking 'Boo hoo, poor little radiologist with their tired eyes, aw diddums'. But visual fatigue is a strong part of feeling knackered. I am no shrinking violet but can genuinely feel wiped out after a day at work despite having barely moved. Tiredness is a strong determinant of making mistakes. So, for patient safety reasons, you don't want a visually tired radiologist.

How dark should reporting rooms be then? A modern medical-grade computer monitor pumps out around 350 candelas per square meter. Candela (cd) is the SI unit of luminosity. It is also called candlepower as 1 cd is roughly the light emitted by one candle—one of those rare occasions where SI units vaguely make sense. 350 cd/m^2 is the equivalent of an old school 40 W incandescent bulb, like early evening light.

Computer monitors are ten times less bright than the old-school light boxes. They had to be bright so as to penetrate the dark film. But such was the brightness of these light boxes that it was like the therapy given for Seasonal Affective Disorder, possibly explaining why radiologists were a lot more genial back then.

Radiology reporting rooms are generally darker than early evening light. It isn't all about deterring visitors. Although if an interloper sticks their head round the door and can only make out vague shapes in the darkness, they then tend to just leave without another word. Which is a win if you really don't want to be

P. McCoubrie, *The Rules of Radiology*, https://doi.org/10.1007/978-3-030-65229-6_48

disturbed. The darkness is, in essence, a do not disturb sign. It isn't a primary goal. A physical sign would be more effective, to be honest.

Radiologists and darkness have been associated since Röntgen first discovered the sainted X-ray. He noticed a fluorescent glow from a barium platinocyanide-coated screen when his cathode ray tube was switched on. If he'd had the lights on, he wouldn't have noticed and they'd not have been discovered. Radiology was born out of darkness on that fateful Friday in November 1895.

Fluoroscopy and film radiography dominated radiology for ninety years until CT, MRI and ultrasound came along. Fluoroscopy demanded darkness. The fluoroscopic screens weren't very good, you see. They were so feeble that it had to be pitch black to see the image at all. So dark, in fact, that radiologists had to dark-adapt for at least fifteen minutes before they used the machine. Dark conditions allow the rod cells in the retina to produce high levels of photopigment, allowing a degree of night vision.

This is all well before my time but before a fluoroscopy session, radiologists would put on specific very dark red goggles to allow their eyes to adapt to the darkness whilst still in normal light. The rod cells of the eye are rather insensitive to red light. So red goggles allow dark adaption whilst still being able to see. Once in the dark room, the goggles came off. Except these goggles were quite sinister even then; very much the mad scientist look.

There is an apparently true tale of a radiologist who wore these goggles outside in public. He regularly walked up St Michael's Hill in Bristol going from the Bristol Royal Infirmary to the old Children's Hospital. He wanted to dark adapt prior to a fluoroscopy session. Apparently someone thought it'd be a terrible wheeze to ring the police and warn them of a strange man walking around with red goggles on. Fortunately the radiologist saw the funny side of it. But he stopped wearing them outdoors thereafter.

Radiology and darkness have remained synonymous despite fluoroscopy having improved immeasurably. Not only that but radiologists continue to embrace the concept of working in the dark. They aren't embarrassed by it; they think it is quite cool. If a clinician thinks they are insulting a radiologist by calling them a vampire, the radiologist laps it up. The clinician thinks ghoulish undead, the radiologist thinks powerful being with irresistible charm. Enticing junior doctors to become radiologists is known as 'calling them to the Dark Side'.

As well as being dark, radiology reporting rooms have to be quiet. Deathly quiet. Understandably, really. Radiologists are trying to concentrate and they don't want distractions. Distracted radiologists lose focus and make mistakes. These days you'll often see radiologist with headphones or ear buds. Sometimes they are't listening to anything just blocking out noise so that they can concentrate. Headphones are, again, a subtle sort of 'do not disturb' sign.

You might think that listening to music whilst reporting is a distraction. However, there isn't any good evidence one way or the other. Some radiologists prefer silence and some prefer background music. Playing music out loud in the reporting room is an absolute no–no. As are open-backed headphones that transmit a tinny beat. What sort of music do radiologists listen to? I could suggest a few albums, perhaps Dark Side of the Moon by Pink Floyd or Back in Black by AC/ DC? Anything by The Darkness also works well.

Sitting alone in quiet dark rooms for long periods of time is, if you think about it, not very doctor-y. As a cliche it couldn't be further from the dashing white coat-clad surgeon or besuited owlish physician with steepled fingers. It does make others think radiologists are reclusive, introverted and antisocial. This couldn't be far from the truth. I am definitely extroverted. Most of my colleagues are gregarious. There are a few oddballs but that is true of any profession.

One downside of working in a windowless room is the winter time. The further from the equator you live, the worse this is. Radiologists arrive at work whilst it is dark, are stuck in a dark room all day and it is dark when they go home. In the Northern Hemisphere, the period from November to January allows many radiologists to only see daylight at weekends. By February, a radiologist's complexion has gone from the normal pasty hue to an unhealthy translucency. By early March, vampire isn't a bad description.

Anyway, back to the need for dark reporting rooms. I need to talk to you about 'subjective contrast'. It is a grossly neglected topic, virtually unknown outside of radiology circles. Many radiologists don't explicitly know it either. You will be aware of the notion of contrast or differing tones on a greyscale. A radiologist needs to be able to see these differing shades to be able to distinguish diseases on an x-ray or scan.

The more contrast there is, the easier the disease is to see. For example, kidney stones are easy see on CT as they are so dense compared to the soft tissues. But some are devilishly hard. Take tumours in the liver, pancreas or kidney. Very tricky to spot as they are near-as-dammit the same grey as the organ that they are in. The aim of giving various sorts of contrast media is that increasing contrast can make diseases easier to see. Radiologists want inherent contrast on the image and will use any trick to make the disease process stand-out like a light bulb. But the contrast inherent in an image cannot always be seen if the viewing conditions are not optimal.

You will be aware that the human eye can see a large range of differing greys. Under ideal circumstances the eye can immediately differentiate around 1000 different greys. Which is roughly 10-bits ($2^{10} = 1024$ levels). This is a lot. With dark adaptation and pupil dilatation, this improves further. But viewing conditions are usually not ideal. This is where the subjective bit comes in.

I often hear clinicians say 'Cor, your computer screens are so much better than ours'. I usually smile and ask, 'Do you turn the light off to look at the pictures?' To which they normally look mildly bewildered. I point to their screen positioned next to a window or directly under a light. They still don't get it. I patiently explain but the screens never move, the curtains are never drawn and the lights stay on.

Ideal viewing circumstances are a very bright image in a black room. That is it. It is very simple. The brighter the image, the easier it is to distinguish differing greys. The darker the room, the more contrast you can see. An optimal viewing environment has a very high ratio of image brightness to ambient light. The ambient light to prevent eye strain has to be balanced against loss of subjective contrast. Hence a radiologist reporting with the light on is an embarrassment; an ignoramus deserved of contempt.

Similarly, a clinician visiting a radiology department must be mindful of this. If they walk into my reporting room then they mustn't complain about how dark it is. It is my darkness; mine, you hear? And, whatever they do, they must not turn the bleedin' light on. If they do, I will throttle them with their own stethoscope.

Chapter 49
Rule #49 / / Don't Touch The Screens

Not with greasy fingers, never ever with pens. The dirtier the screen you'll tolerate, the sloppier a radiologist you are.

—

The computer screen is the work-bench of a diagnostic radiologist. My PACS monitor is the equivalent of the physician's examination couch or the surgeon's operating table. Actually, screens are more important than that. An examination couch is a minor luxury. Give a surgeon anything pointy and sharp and they'd make do. Whereas I am hamstrung without a screen. The screen is everything.

A modern medical computer screen is liquid crystal-based and hence fragile. So they have a protective layer over the front. You'd have thought they'd use toughened glass and some of the very expensive ones do. Most don't. This frontispiece is usually fairly soft plastic and marks easily. It is also difficult to polish and nearly impossible to replace. Scratch it and you've just ruined a £2 k bit of kit.

It used to be the same with x-ray film. The touching thereof was also *verboten*. There was only thing that was allowed to touch the film and this was the chinagraph pencil (a grease pencil for US readers). Slightly odd, if you think about it, drawing all over the film with coloured wax. But it rubs off fairly easily and leaves no residue. This all changed overnight when the UK kissed goodbye to film in 2006 through a national digitisation project. Indeed, my hospital doesn't have a single light box. Although, oddly, we do still have a box of chinagraph pencils.

Of all the things to point with, pens must never go near a screen. People think it is more hygienic or clever to point with a pen. But even with the nib retracted, pens are alarmingly scratchy. Whilst I can allow a finger up to five cm or so from the screen, I cannot allow a pen within a metre. A pen approaching a screen is like someone waving a knife near the paintwork of my car. Most people's depth perception is less than perfect and the unthinkable happens regularly. The sound of a pen even lightly tapping on a screen makes me flinch.

The only item that can be pointed at a screen with is a dedicated blunt-ended pointer. These extensible devices are under-rated devices for teaching. I've long fancied one as they have a nerdish chic. Plus, if used correctly, they can be a fantastically comedic device. If you don't believe me, the master of the pointer is my favourite radiological anti-hero, Dr Alan Statham, the radiologist character in the TV series *Green Wing*.

Given the primacy of screens, their expense and fragility then you'd naturally assume they are handled gently, have regular organised maintenance and frequent cleaning. But no. They are installed and forgotten. Dirty and lightly damaged screens are therefore quite common in radiology departments. Most hospitals will happily invest £1-2 k in a screen but not £2 every few months for a packet of screen wipes. This means that well-meaning individuals make misguided cleaning attempts with a general purpose wipe. These leave faint soapy smears that actually make matters worse.

PACS monitors show up fingerprints and other mucky smears quiet beautifully. Most screens are the same. It was only relatively recently that it became normal for smart phones and tablet computers to not have a fingerprint problem. The early versions of these needed a regular polish as fingerprints gradually obscured the screen. Oil in these fingerprints has a different refractive property to glass and bends the light differently, causing a focal blur. Most touchscreens now have an oleophobic coating so the oil stays on your finger and the glass feels slick to touch.

There is a very real risk with a dirty screen. Many is the time that I had just been on the verge of diagnosing a subtle lung cancer only to realise that the 'lesion' can be wiped away with an exploratory finger. The more the fingerprints, the more blurred the image. Blur is fine if you want to give cinematic heroines a glowing complexion, like the vaseline-coated filters used on Ingrid Bergman in *Casablanca*. But obscuring detail is the very opposite of what a radiologist needs.

You will know the fascination that small children have with pressing their face and hands on clean glass. You may remember doing it yourself. Maybe you did it recently—I won't judge you if you have. The joy from this doesn't fade with age. There seems to be something pleasant about the cool feeling and novelty of the invisible barrier. Particularly if you aren't the one cleaning it afterwards.

The same is true of clinicians. Well, I will admit they don't press their face against my PACS monitor. Not even the most infantile orthopaedic surgeon does this. I did hear a rumour that they had to replace all the computer monitors in the orthopaedic department. The IT department couldn't clean all the crayon off the screens, you see. This aside, clinicians cannot help stabbing their fingers at the abnormality on the screen when discussing it.

Incidentally, the marks left by fingers are fascinating. They are predominantly formed from natural protective skin oils. This has the medical name of sebum, from the Latin for 'grease'. Sebum is a mix of triglycerides, waxy esters, fatty acids and squalene. It is produced by the sebaceous glands of which we each have several million. They are everywhere apart from the palms of the hands and soles of the feet. The fingertips have few sebaceous glands. Most of the sebum in a fingerprint is actually from the hair or face, transferred after touching. So a fingerprint on a screen is effectively the same as someone having squished their nose on it. Which is both alarming and disgusting.

Sebum from your nose, incidentally, contains a higher proportion of squalene. Squalene is a durable oil that can act as a lubricant and a polish. Indeed, my grandfather used to shine the bowl of his tobacco pipe on his nose. Which is both alarming and disgusting but logical, if you think about it. The other major source of squalene in nature is shark liver extract. I would contend that your schnozzle is an more environmentally-friendly source of lubricants than poor Mr Shark's liver. Also this handy source of lubricant is literally right in front of you at all times.

One of the first things I teach new radiology trainees is not to touch the screens. I highlight this important cultural step shortly after their transit to the Dark Side. Breaking this habit early is important. I stop short of slapping hands away from the screen or rewarding them for not touching the screen with a pellet of food. But there is no negotiation on this. This is an absolute rule. I insist on it.

Beyond keeping the screen clean, there is another very good reason for insisting that young radiologists sit on their hands. Once gesticulation is forbidden then the neophytes have to use words to describe the location of the thing they are describing. Which is what radiologists do in their written reports every day. The common phrase that radiology trainers employ is, 'Imagine you are describing it to me on the telephone'. Accurately describing where something is located is half the trick of this radiology lark.

There is a wider issue about dirt and messy working environments. Some reporting areas can become horrifically cluttered, usually with bits of paper dominating the debris. To the casual observer, it looks like a dog has attacked a book and no one cleared it up. Except that every scrap has been written on. Numerous spidery scripts indicate that several radiologists are to blame, scribbling on anything that came to hand.

Most PACS stations are flanked by a number of textbooks in varying degrees of disassembly. Typically this is an early version of the Keat's Atlas of Normal Variants (a.k.a The Book of Missed Fractures). This usually lies in bits due to a broken spine, which is ironic, if you think about it.

Another particular bugbear is dirty cups, often several generations of them around a shared workspace. Some colleagues have breathtakingly poor hygiene standards, where the weeks-old milky coffee remnant acts as some form of culture medium. Woe betide anyone that accidentally knocks them over and spills the primordial soup within. I looked in one of these cups just recently and I swear something moved in it. I think I witnessed evolution in action.

Apart from the potential health and safety risks, such jumbled chaos distracts from the task in hand. It is also dispiriting. Disarray doesn't exactly lift the soul. Put these all together and you've got a pretty poor working environment. The sad thing is that such cluttered conditions are commonplace. I'm astonished by what some radiologists will put up with.

A messy reporting room is messy because cleanliness is not a priority for radiologists. Unfortunately this mess makes radiologists look like slothful degenerates.

All the effort expended on inculcating a gleaming professional reputation is utterly undone by a reporting room that looks like a bomb has just gone off.

Radiologists should smarten their act up and revel in the benefits. They should pretend that their screen is the Mona Lisa—nothing touches it, nothing comes near. Radiologist should declutter ruthlessly; adopt a zero tolerance policy for mess in shared workspaces. And for God's sake, won't someone wash those cups up?

Chapter 50
Rule #50 / / Error Is Inherent To Radiology

Get used to it. The images are subjective. Every cancer starts really, really small. The human body is really, really complex. See Rule #51.

—

If you were to throw a ball gently up in the air then most of us would be able to catch it again. In fact most of us would be confident of catching it. If you throw it up often enough times, however, eventually you will drop it. Admittedly with practice and focus you'd probably drop it less often. But everyone drops easy catches from time to time, even professional sports players who are paid good money to catch balls.

Obviously certain catches are more difficult. We can't all be Andrew Strauss, the then English Cricket Captain, who dismissed Adam Gilchrist in the 2005 fourth Ashes Test Match by flinging himself through the air like Superman to hold onto an improbable and brilliant one-handed catch (Fig. 50.1). This said, anyone who undergoes specific and prolonged training has an increased chance of taking such catches.

Certain catches are impossible. The ball comes so fast that you cannot react. Or you run and leap like a salmon but can't get near it. You can practice and practice until your fingers bleed but it won't make a difference—you only take these catches rarely and only then through luck or bizarre circumstances. No one blames you if you miss it. The ball is simply not there to catch.

Of course the parallel I am drawing is between dropping a catch and error in radiology. Just like a sports player, a highly trained radiologist makes fewer mistakes. Hence radiologists should seek to continuously improve their abilities. It is also true that perfectly well-trained radiologist will occasionally metaphorically drop the ball. They will make a mistake for no particular reason. The diagnostic task was not unduly difficult. The radiologist was alert, focussed and sober. There is no way on God's fair planet that they'd normally fluff this up.

© The Author(s), under exclusive license to Springer Nature Switzerland AG 2021
P. McCoubrie, *The Rules of Radiology*, https://doi.org/10.1007/978-3-030-65229-6_50

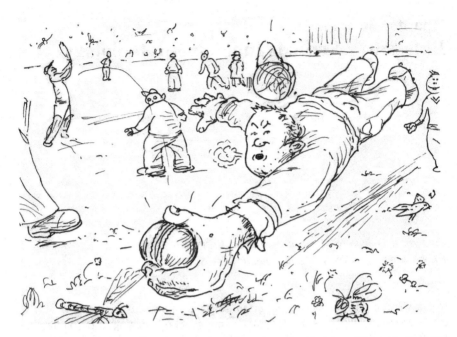

Fig. 50.1 "Andrew Strauss's brilliant one-handed catch to dismiss Adam Gilchrist in the 2005 Ashes series"

You might think that this is rare. Highly trained individuals don't muck up very often. This is where the analogy falls apart. Radiology isn't catching a ball. It is more complex than a simple psychomotor task. There are four main things that can go wrong: observer error; error in interpretation, failure to give guidance and failure to communicate in a timely and appropriate manner. Failure of just one of these factors can result in error.

Observer error is the most common of these. The radiologist fails to spot the abnormality. Many fine words have been written about failure of perception but I think it is simple: to err is human. Even the best radiological eye is fallible; the best radiological brain can misjudge. There is a randomness and statistical inevitability to diagnostic errors just as there is in procedural radiology (see Rule #32).

To me it is a minor miracle that radiologists see so much and miss so little. When I was a medical student I was in awe of radiologists who could look at a film and see things that twenty other people in the room could not. I am now that radiologist who can see things that others cannot. I'm both proud of this and also mildly baffled. I say baffled as I cannot explain it easily. I just can. Visual expertise isn't easy to explain.

Misclassification is probably the second most common error. This is where the radiologist sees the abnormality but mistakes it for something else. It's a difficult topic but, as we discussed in Rule #47, radiology has the science of uncertainty at its very heart. Radiologists will not stop misclassifying any time soon. Plus, as we will see in Rule #66, over-calling normality is just as much of an error as under-calling abnormality.

Communication errors are less common. Several things can go wrong. Sometimes error arises where the English language is tortured to the point of unreadability (see Rule #23). Sometimes the report is unreadably long and important findings are hidden (see Rule #24). Sometimes error arises through vagueness and ambiguity (see Rule #29).

There are other ways in which the report can fail. Radiologists are expected to give advice in their reports, particularly to non-specialists on urgent issues. Which sounds fair enough but relies on the radiologist knowing how a huge range of serious conditions should be managed. Which isn't a radiology thing, really. So it isn't surprising that radiologists sometimes slip up here.

Although no one tells you this on day one of radiology school, it is the legal responsibility of radiologists to ensure the report reaches the correct person in a timely manner. A radiologist's duty extends beyond clicking the 'verify' button. Hand-delivering reports on a silver salver is a little much but there is no doubt-some clinicians would love this, particularly if the radiologist bowed as they did so. In the real world, efficient secretaries and agreed urgent communication protocols are the only answer to this.

Given these many possibilities of error, it would be strange indeed to be always in the right. The modern expectation is not to miss anything at all. This is a bit unfair but perhaps is an indictment of our times that society is not more enlightened and routinely seeks to apportion blame, to scandalise and to dispute any error.

On the other hand, I find it inspiring that attitudes to error within radiology have changed so much in my professional lifetime. Only a generation ago, error was frowned on and routinely swept under the carpet. Now it is a respected field of study. Many radiology journal pages and many beads of radiological sweat have been dedicated to the study of radiological error.

Most of these papers have been published in the last twenty years. Some studies have estimated error rates for complex tasks at up 40%, usually also noting that experts have better performance. This is fine until you realise that most of these papers are a flimsily-disguised exercise in self-congratulation and protectionism. It usually turns out that 'experts' are classified as people curiously similar to the authors. Hence everyone else is unhelpfully painted as dangerously incompetent and shouldn't dabble unless they become more like the authors.

For more routine radiological tasks, studies have unearthed a baseline error rate that doesn't seem to drop below around 3–5%. Although an accuracy of 95–97% is not too shabby, it isn't perfect. There are those who say that patients should be warned about this and be given written information on the matter. I personally don't think it would help—folk are numb to legal disclaimers these days and the majority are ignored. They can sow confusion and certainly don't stop complaints.

There is a particular controversy worthy of discussion. This is deciding if, in fact, an error has been made. Was it a catchable catch? Or was it uncatchable? It isn't always easy to decide as mistakes look easy in retrospect (see Rule #65). It is why radiologists often called errors 'discrepancies' as they are either just disagree-ments of opinion or disagreements about whether or not an error happened.

This discussion is at the heart of many medico-legal cases where liability and negligence are crucial. Although radiologists often reassure each other by claiming the original abnormality was impossible to see. Whilst crucial in the eye of the Law, it doesn't help radiologists learn if they are shamed or made to feel guilty. Retrospective judgement impedes learning from mistakes. It's an complex issue and I will discuss it more fully in Rule #51.

Another controversy is the assumption that radiologists who make errors must be below average. Of course all radiologists make errors (see Rule #74) so this isn't always true. It is also based on a misunderstanding of the distribution of expertise amongst radiologists. Most would expect that this normally distributed (i.e. Gaussian) and if you plotted it on a graph, you'd make a bell-curve.

Except this isn't true. Expert performance normally follows a Paretian distribu-tion, named after Italian polymath Vilfredo Pareto. The shape of this is an expo-nential curve. Most radiologists are high-functioning and there is little to separate them. They exist on gently sloping right hand part of the curve. The left hand side of the curve is a steep tail of performance, featuring a minority of radiologists of varying degrees of incompetence. This distribution follows the rough 80:20 rule; where the bottom 20% of radiologists make 80% of the mistakes.

It is a controversial theory but there is ample evidence that this is true. Plus it has connotations. One way of reducing error is to simply the sack the bottom 20% of radiologists. Furthermore 80% can be left alone to safely get on with it. The major difficulty is knowing where the individual radiologist sits on this curve. It is difficult to judge this accurately and full of hazards for anyone who tries to do it. Plus competence is very specific. It is quite possible to be hopeless at scanning the groin but be a world-expert in the scrotum, a structure only 5 cm away (see Rule #93).

The important message about the inevitability of error is not one of hopeless-ness and dread. The message is actually one of tempered hope. Yes, radiologists will fluff up from time to time and they need resilience (see Rule #5) but error can be mitigated by high professional standards and robust systems of work.

Appendix

Rule #51 / / Savour mistakes

And near misses too. Even the best radiologists can make the worst mistakes. You cannot know it all. But everyone can learn. See Rules #39 and #50

Rule #52 / / Don't rush a report

Clinicians bizarrely expect it instantly. The more complex the scan, the sicker the patient, the closer they crowd you. Dispel them with 'You can have the wrong report now or the correct report in 15 minutes'

Rule #53 / / Never wake a patient up

If they are sound asleep, they don't need a scan right now. Sleep is good for ill people. However, probably wise to double-check they are actually asleep and not moribund.

Rule #54 / / Know about esoterica

If you hear hoof beats and see stripes, it could be a zebra. There are so many rare conditions that it is common to have at least one of them in the hospital. See Rule #39.

Rule #55 / / Doctors aren't porters

If you let them just 'drop off a form' and leave without another word then you are doing them, you and the patient a disservice.

P. McCoubrie, *The Rules of Radiology*, https://doi.org/10.1007/978-3-030-65229-6

Rule #56 / / Don't shoot the messenger

It isn't the poor newbie medical houseman's fault that the 'surgeons want a CT before they see the patient'. Instead of ripping them a new orifice, save your ire for the original miscreant. See Rules #36 and #37

Rule #57 / / Question 'protocols'

If the major reason for a scan is due to 'the protocol', ask to see it 'for my education'. The protocol in question usually either doesn't exist or states exactly the contrary.

Rule #58 / / Don't be a hairdresser

Hairdressers never say 'you don't need a hair cut'. Question the motives of those who are paid per scan, especially when they recommend expensive additional studies.

Rule #59 / / Prognostication is not an indication

If someone is so ill that they are not fit for a haircut then a scan isn't going to change anything. It is wasting everyone's time. See Rules #15 and #64.

Rule #60 / / Beware of Mr Twitchy

If a patient can't stay still, abandon it straight away. Get them back another time. Otherwise you get asked to interpret a twitchogram. And that never ends well.

Rule #61 / / Always look at the scout image or localisers

That 10cm RCC isn't on the sag T2. And that basal lung cancer isn't on the volume dataset. Ignore them at your medico-legal peril.

Rule #62 / / Dictate considerately

If a secretary 6 rooms away can clearly transcribe your every word, you should probably speak a little more quietly. You are also probably irritating your colleagues beyond belief.

Rule #63 / / Don't scan instead of talking

Resist pressure to omit clinical discussion. Talking is cheap, quick and can avoid scans altogether. It also has relatively few serious side effects.

Rule #64 / / Never scan the dying

It is highly distressing, undignified and tantamount to assault. No amount of diagnostic electromagnetic waves will stop Mother Nature. See Rule #59.

Rule #65 / / Don't be a smart arse

Scans often only become a waste of time after you've done them. It's easy to be wise with hindsight: only a facile radiologist does this.

Rule #66 / / False positives are errors too

Over-calling is as equal a sin to under-calling. If you can't report a CXR without asking for a CT, you need to take a long hard look at yourself. See Rules #29, #50 and #51.

Rule #67 / / Vetting requests is worthwhile

If you let other people do it for you (or don't do it at all), you cannot complain about unjustified scans or scrambled clinical reasoning. Man up and JFDI.

Rule #68 / / Be a holistic radiologist

Look at the whole image not just your area of interest. You may be the cleverest spinal radiologist since the Earth cooled but missing a 7cm AAA on MRI L-spine is never clever.

Rule #69 / / Radiology is extrapolating from a screen grab

If life is a box set and illness is a single episode, radiologists are left to infer the plot from a single screen shot. This explains why radiology is so damned difficult sometimes

Rule #70 / / Coffee should be taken black

Coffee is the lifeblood of radiology, our dominant fuel source. Thus the Bean should be treated with total respect. Never ever syrup, sugar with caution, warm milk only in extenuating circumstances

Rule #71 / / Radiology reporting is like playing golf in the dark

Your swing may be sound but you have little idea of where the ball lands. Clinico-pathological feedback is a radiological imperative. Without it, all confidence is misplaced

Rule #72 / / Never report 'no change'

It is a supremely unhelpful radiology report. It is only permitted in one specific circumstance - when reporting an x-ray of a child looking for swallowed coins

Rule #73 / / Always report in date order

The oldest studies get done first, irrespective of their complexity, image quality or indication. Cherry picking is the mark of a lazy and selfish radiologist

Rule #74 / / Beware the radiologist with a zero % error rate

It either means they are (a) perfect (b) doing no work or (c) being dishonest. Given (a) is impossible and (b) is unlikely it means that (c) must be true

Rule #75 / / Interventional radiologists don't need to care

Technical ability always trumps empathy and communication skills. The heart of an IR doesn't need to be in the right place but their lines should be

Rule #76 / / Radiology should be fun

Radiologists are medicine's dolphins, frolicking in its warm waters. If it doesn't feel like fun then you need a holiday. Failing that, move to a hospital where you are valued

Rule #77 / / There is no such thing as a 'naturally gifted' radiologist

Natural talent is a myth. Show me a talented radiologist and I'll show you some-one who works their socks off. Show me a duffer and I'll show you some a radiologist who opens neither books nor journals.

Rule #78 / / Introduce yourself

Just because you are a radiologist doesn't mean you are above common courtesy. Greet patients and staff by turning to them, smiling, fixing eye contact and proffering a brief but firm handshake whilst saying "Hello, my name is ...". Do this every time. Especially the last bit

Rule #79 / / Trust in chronometry

Those that take twice the time to report their scans are half as good. The corollary isn't true. Those that take half the time to report their scans are also half as good.

Rule #80 / / Ignore 3D recons

No self-respecting radiologist would ever use them for primary diagnosis. And, no, they aren't interesting or clever either. They are mere pretty baubles to keep the surgeons happy

Rule #81 / / AI is overhyped

Whenever anyone says AI will replace radiologists, you have my personal permission to beat them with their own shoes

Rule #82 / / Do the simple things well & often

If you are courteous, honest, well-presented, organised, methodical and work with a slick team in a clean environment, then you are >90% of the way there. Heroics are rarely necessary and paradoxically unhelpful

Rule #83 / / Show yourself

An invisible colleague is an annoying colleagueBeavering away in a quiet corner mustn't be the default. If you can't be found easily, you aren't doing your fair share. Step out of the shadows and pull your weight.

Rule #84 / / Don't criticise colleagues

It is unwarranted - they are usually trying their hardest. It is unhelpful - a knife in the back helps no one. It is destructive - it sours relations. A good radiologist leads by example and encourages others

Rule #85 / / You can only eat one breakfast

Quality of life & happiness barely increase as income rises >£50k. And yet monetary squabbles are a common cause of rancour between radiologists. Rise above this. If you are in it for the money, you are in the wrong trade

Rule #86 / / You Will Learn to Hate VR

Yes, yes, yes; voice recognition has brought some benefits. However, it turns most radiologists into expensive secretaries. And nothing in your working life is quite so annoying, quite so often

Rule #87 / / Dress smartly

The vogue for dressing down is to be resisted. You are a doctor, dammit; dress like one. The less formal your clothes, the less respect you'll get. If you look like a scruffy overgrown teen don't complain when you are treated like one

Rule #88 / / Focus on the gaps

Time taken to report a scan or perform a procedure is irrelevant. It is a statistic, not a quality measure. Some scans take longer. Some people take longer. The time wasted before and between scans or procedures should be the focus

Rule #89 / / Eminence doesn't equal sense

Confidence wears off slower than skill in the aged radiologist. Grey hair and notoriety doesn't mean infallibility. Often the opposite.

Rule #90 / / Sloppiness is infectious

People inherently cut corners. Sometimes it is because they work in a crap system. Sometimes it is because they are lazy. Don't just shrug complacently - do something. The standard you walk past is the standard you accept

Rule #91 / / Never assume relationships

An attractive 20-something with a frail octogenarian are usually grandchild & grandparent. But the one time you voice this, you can guarantee that they'll be married. Avoid foot-in-mouth disease:- always ask

Rule #92 / / 'Order Comms' must be loathed

First, no radiologist should let themselves be 'ordered' to do anything. Second, one-way transmission prevents clinicoradiological discussion. Last, it denies a key perk of the job as there is no physical card to rip up

Rule #93 / / Don't blame the 'bad apple'

Improvement by removing a 'bad apple' from the barrel is a fallacy. It is virtually always a barrel issue. It is just that apples are easier to blame. An enlightened radiologist blames neither: they learn, they improve

Rule #94 / / Structured reporting is overblown

Structure in reports is always good but structured reports aren't always good. Such reports are over-long and mind-numbingly bland; the antithesis of a readable report. And an unreadable report is a dangerous report

Rule #95 / / Beware pixel-squeezers

Some radiologists will try to convince you of the significance of tiny isolated abnormalities only a few pixels across. Or worse, minor variations in the shade of faux-colour. You can safely ignore them; they are making it up

Rule #96 / / Embrace Productivity

Attempts to improve productivity are normally just harder cracks of the same whip. This achieves nothing apart from burnout. But looking at ways of achieving the same goal more easily and effectively indicates enlightenment

Rule #97 / / Be a kind boss

Radiologists can find themselves in leadership positions, often accidentally. Be the boss you would like to have had. You can be decisive, effective and yet remain kind. Whereas inhuman autocrats are toxic, ineffective and hated.

Rule #98 / / Embrace Diversity

Great departments are staffed by radiologists of varying age, gender, race, culture & personality. This serves both referrers & patients well. But coherence is vital. It falls flat if you aren't all pulling in the same direction

Rule #99 / /Look After Yourself

You cannot escape the anxieties incident to professional life. But when going the extra mile becomes the norm, you are on the road to burnout. A burnt out radiologist is tragic: tragic for themselves, tragic for their patients

Rule #100 / / It's all about the patient

It isn't about you, the referrer, the institution or the health system. It never was and never will be. Each and every act of a radiologist should directly benefit the patient. Lose this principle and you lose everything

Index

Printed in the United States
by Baker & Taylor Publisher Services